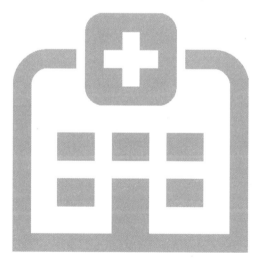

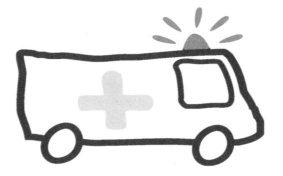

간호영어 병원영어

Hospital English

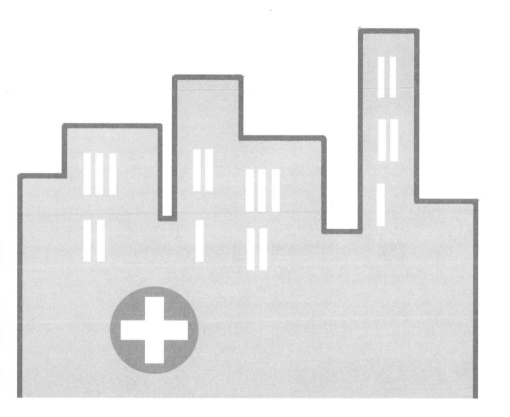

병원에서 의료인들이 가장 많이 사용하는
간결한 임상 영어들을 담았습니다.

Part I : Hospital Ward
제 1부 : 병동에서

Part II : Hospital Departments Services
제 2부 : 병원 전문과목별 서비스 (외래 및 분과)

Part III : Health Check Up, Radiology,
            Laboratory Room and Administration
제 3부 : 건강 검진, 방사선과, 임상병리과 및 원무과

프롤로그

국가 간의 경계가 사라지면서

외국인 환자들이 국내병원에서 진료를 받는 경우가 많아지고 있습니다.

이렇게 글로벌화 해지는 사회적 변화에 따라

의료인들의 국제화된 감각이나

기본적인 의사소통이 필요한 시기입니다.

몇 년간 의사들이 보는 의협신문에

의료인들을 위한 진료영어를 연재하였고,

자주 꺼내어 볼 수 있게 책으로도 발간하였습니다.

하지만 임상영어 위주이다 보니

간호사나 병원의 각 분야 의료인들이 사용하기에는

미흡한 부분이 많았습니다.

그래서 진료 이외의 시간을 이용하여,

영어에 능숙하지 않은 의료인들을 위해,

병원의 병동이나 외래 또는 각 전문파트에서 쓸 수 있는

실용적인 병원에서의 간결한 영어 표현들을,

'간호영어 병원영어'란 제목으로 모아 보았습니다.

아무쪼록 이 책을 필요로 하는 독자들에게

작은 도움이 되었으면 하는 바램입니다.

2017년 2월 임창석 씀

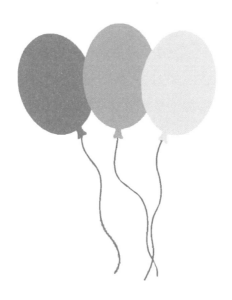

We are open to the experience

of the present moment in the hospital.

목 차

Part I : Hospital Ward (제 1부 : 병동에서)

Part II : Hospital Departments Services
(제 2부 : 병원 전문과목별 서비스 – 외래 및 분과)

Part III : Health Check Up, Radiology,

Laboratory Room and Administration

(제 3부 : 건강 검진, 방사선과, 임상병리과 및 원무과)

N : Nurse P : Patient or Patient's Family A : Administrator

Part I : Hospital Ward

제 1부 : 병동에서

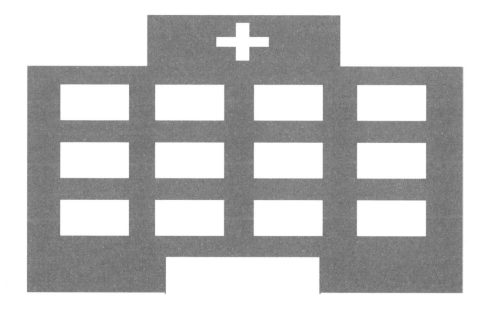

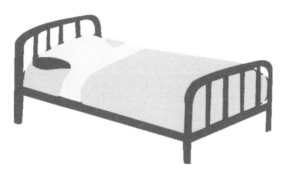

1. 입원환자 맞이하기

Very Useful Expressions

1. Hi. Are you Mr. (Mrs. Miss) –?
   안녕하세요, –씨인가요?
2. I'll be taking care of you in this ward.
   이 병동에서 당신을 간호할 것입니다.
3. I am one of the nurses taking care of you here.
   여기서 당신을 간호할 간호사 중 한 명입니다.
4. I'll be doing day shifts
   and looking after you for the next few days.
   며칠 동안 낮에 근무하며 당신을 돌보게 될 것입니다.
5. We are currently preparing your room,
   please wait a minute.
   지금 당신의 방을 준비 중이니, 조금만 기다려 주십시오.
6. Your room will be ready soon.
   당신의 방은 곧 준비가 될 것입니다.
7. You have to wait until other patient is discharged.
   다른 환자가 퇴원하기 전까지 기다리셔야 합니다.
8. You have to wait until the room is cleaned.
   방 청소가 끝날 때까지 기다리셔야 합니다.
9. It will take about 20 minutes.
   20분 정도 걸립니다.

10. I'd like to ask some questions prior to admission.

입원하기 전에 몇 가지를 물어보겠습니다.

12. What health problems are you being admitted for?

어떤 건강상 문제로 입원하셨나요?

13. What brings you in?

무슨 일로 입원하셨죠?

14. Once admitted to the hospital,

we will be taking care of you.

일단 병원에 입원하시면 우리가 당신을 돌보아 줄 것입니다.

15. You need to put on the patient's identity bracelet.

환자 신원확인 팔찌를 착용하셔야 합니다.

16. I'll show you around the ward.

병실 주변을 가르쳐 드리겠습니다.

입원환자를 대할 때는 Hi, Hello, Hi there, Hi dear 등을

가장 많이 사용하고, 환자의 연령이나 상태, 상황에 따라

Good morning (afternoon, evening). Good to see you.

Nice to meet you. 등의 표현들을 적절하게 사용한다.

환자에게 자신이 담당 간호사라는 말할 때는

I'll be one of the nurses taking care of you.

I'll be taking care of you in this ward.

I'll be looking after you today.

I am your nurse on this shift. I'll be taking care of you today.

I'm taking care of you here. 등

여러 가지를 사용할 수 있고,

환자에게 며칠 동안 낮에 근무한다는 표현은

I'll be on shift during the day for the next few days.

I'll be doing day shifts for the next few days. 로 할 수 있다.

환자에게 어떤 문제로 입원하게 되었는가 물어보려면,

What health problems are you being admitted for?

What symptoms made you to be admitted to the hospital?

Why are you being admitted today?

Tell me why you came in? What seems to be the problem?

What brings you in today?

등을 사용한다.

Conversation

P : Hello. I am supposed to be admitted to this hospital.

안녕하세요. 이 병원에 입원하기로 되어있는 환자인데요.

N : Hi, you must be Mr. Jones.

안녕하세요. 아마도 존스씨 맞으시죠?

P : Yes, I am. Dr. Kim told me that hospital stay is necessary

for treatment.

네 그렇습니다. 김선생님이 치료를 받으려면 입원이 필요하다고 말씀을

하시더군요.

N : Nice to meet you.

만나서 반갑습니다.

I am a nurse looking after you in this ward.

저는 이 병동에서 당신을 간호할 간호사입니다.

Did you come with your family?

가족들과 함께 오셨나요?

P : No. I came alone.

아뇨. 혼자 왔습니다.

N : OK. Put your luggage on the floor right next to the nurse station
until your room is ready.

알겠습니다. 당신의 방이 준비될 때까지 짐은 간호사 스테이션 바로
옆 바닥에 놓아주십시오.

We are currently preparing your room.

지금 당신의 방을 준비 중입니다.

This may take time.

이것은 시간이 좀 걸릴 수 있습니다.

P : No problem.

알겠습니다.

You look very young to be a nurse.

간호사라고 보기에는 아주 젊으시군요.

N : That's nice to hear.

듣기는 좋은 말이네요.

I've been a nurse for 2 years now.

간호사가 된 지 2년 되었습니다.

P : Really? Don't get me wrong.

그래요? 오해하지 마세요.

I am saying this because I feel a little bit nervous.

조금 긴장이 돼서 이런 말을 하는 것입니다.

N : Don't mind.

신경 쓰지 마세요.

By the way I'd like to ask some questions prior to admission.

그건 그렇고 입원하기 전에 몇 가지 물어보겠습니다.

What problems are you being admitted for?

어떤 문제로 입원하셨나요?

P : I was diagnosed with hepatitis.

간염이라고 진단 받았습니다.

N : When did you first notice your symptoms?

증상을 언제 느끼기 시작했나요?

P : About several months ago.

몇 달 전부터요.

I think, maybe I got it through a tattoo.

아마도 문신하다가 감염된 것 같습니다.

N : Did you ever have jaundice?

황달이 있었던 적이 있나요?

P : No.

아뇨.

N : Don't you feel tired?

피곤하지는 않으세요?

P : I am a little bit tired.

조금 피곤하네요.

And I am hungry.

그리고 배가 고프군요.

N : Are you? Hospital lunch time has passed.

그러세요? 병원 점심시간이 지났네요.

You need to eat outside or have a meal at hospital cafeteria

before admission.

입원하기 전에 밖이나 구내식당에서 식사를 하셔야 되겠네요.

P : Don't mind me.

신경 쓰지 마세요.

I'll eat later.

나중에 먹을게요.

N : OK.

알겠습니다.

P : When will I get to go home?

언제쯤 집에 가게 될까요?

N : Your doctor will explain about that according to the progress of

treatment.

남당선생님이 치료 진행 상황에 따라 그것을 설명해 줄 것입니다.

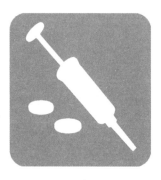

Extra Study

만약 영어에 능숙하지 않을 때, 먼저 꺼낼 수 있는 표현들은

저는 영어를 조금만 할 줄 압니다.

I can speak a little English.

I can speak a bit of English.

영어를 잘 이해하지 못합니다. 천천히 말씀해 주실래요?

I can't understand very well in English.

Could you speak more slowly?

또는

I am not good at English.

Would you mind speaking a bit more slowly?

를 사용하고 대화중 어려움이 있을 때는

뭐라고요? 다시 말해주실래요?

Pardon me? Come again? Excuse me? Say again?

I beg your pardon? Would you say that again?

What was that again?

지금은 영어로 생각이 잘 안 나네요.

It's on the tip of my tongue in English.

I can't recall it right now in English.

I can't think of it at the moment in English.

영어로 잘 표현 하지를 못 합니다.

I can't express myself very well in English.

등을 사용하면 도움이 된다.

2. 입원환자의 증상 및 인적 사항 질문

Very Useful Expressions

1. What seems to be the problem?
   무슨 문제가 있으시죠?

2. Can you tell me your problem?
   무슨 문제가 있으시죠?

3. When did your symptom seem to begin?
   증상이 언제부터 시작되었던 것 같으시나요?

4. How long have you been having your symptoms?
   증상이 있는 지 얼마나 오래 되었죠?

5. How often do you have symptoms?
   얼마나 자주 증상이 생기죠?

6. Where are you having pain?
   어디가 아프시죠?

7. Can you describe your pain on a scale of 0 to 10?
   통증의 정도를 0에서 10까지에서 말해 주실래요?

8. When do you experience your pain?
   언제 통증을 느끼시죠?

9. What kind of pain are you having?
   어떤 통증을 느끼시나요?

10. Can you tell me your full name, please?
    전체 이름을 말씀해 주실래요?

11. What was the name again?

이름이 어떻게 되신다고요?

12. What's your date of birth, please?

생일이 며칠이시죠?

13. Where are you come from?

어느 나라에서 오셨죠?

14. Where do you live?

어디에 사시죠?

15. How old are you?

몇 살이시죠?

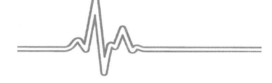

16. Are you married?

결혼은 했나요?

17. How long have you been married?

결혼을 한지 얼마나 되셨어요?

18. How many people are there in your family?

가족이 모두 몇 명이지요?

19. Do you have any children?

아이들이 있나요?

20. What's your occupation?

직업이 무엇이지요?

21. Please read this form and fill it out.

이 양식을 읽어보시고 기입을 해주세요.

무슨 문제가 있으시죠? 또는 어디가 불편하세요? 는

What seems to be the problem? What brings you today?

What's your problem? What's the trouble?

Can you tell me your problem?

Can you describe your symptoms? Can I help you?

Tell me about your symptoms.

Please describe your problems.

I would like to hear about your symptoms.

Would you like to describe your problem?

등을 사용할 수 있고, 증상이 언제 시작이 되었는 지는

When did your symptom seem to begin?

When did your symptom start?

When did you first notice your symptoms?

당신의 증상이 처음 있었을 때를 기억하나요?

Can you remember when your symptom first came on?

증상이 얼마나 되었나요? 는

How long have you had your symptoms?

얼마나 오랫동안 지속되었나요? 는

How long has this been going on?

How long did it last? 등으로 표현한다.

그리고 통증에 대해 질문을 할 때,

갑자기 생겼는지는 Did this pain come on suddenly?

얼마나 자주 나타나는 지는 How often does this pain occur?

How frequently do you have pain? 으로 물어본다.

통증의 특징에 대해서는

당신의 통증 정도를 0에서 10까지의 숫자를 이용하여 말해줄래요?

Describe your pain intensity using a scale of 0 (representing

no pain) to 10 (representing the worst pain imaginable).

그리고 어떤 통증이 느껴지죠? 는

How do you feel your pain?

What does your pain feel like?

What kind of pain are you having?

로 물으며 통증의 양상에 따라

Is it constant or intermittent? Is it sharp or dull?

beating? biting? boring? burning? colicky? cramping? dull?

gripping? heavy? numb? piercing? pressing? prickling?

pulling? sharp? shooting? sore? stabbing? tearing?

throbbing? tingling? twisting? 등으로 표현한다.

결혼 생활에 대해서는 간단하게 Are you married?

아이들이 몇 명 있는 지는? Do you have any children?

How many children do you have?

직업이 무엇인 지는

What do you do for a living? What kind of work do you do?

What business are you in? What's your job?

What's your occupation? What's your work? 이고

이 양식을 천천히 읽어보고 작성을 해서 저희들에게 돌려주세요. 는

Please take the time to read and

fill out this form and return to us. 로 표현한다.

Conversation

N : Hi there, I will take care of you today.

안녕하세요. 제가 오늘 당신을 돌볼 것입니다.

P : Nice to meet you.

만나서 반갑습니다.

N : What would you like me to call you?

제가 무어라 부르면 좋을까요?

May I call you James or would you prefer Mr. Dean?

제임스라고 부를까요? 아니면 미스터 딘이라고 할까요?

P : Both are all right.

둘 다 좋습니다.

N : Where are you come from?

어느 나라에서 오셨죠?

P : USA.

미국에서 왔습니다.

N : Room and bed arrangement is underway.

방과 침대 배치에 대해 조정 중입니다.

You will have to wait a half hour.

30분 정도 기다리셔야 할 것입니다.

P : OK. No problem.

알겠습니다. 괜찮습니다.

N : First of all, let me ask you something.

먼저 몇 가지 물어볼게요.

What seems to be the problem?

무슨 문제가 있으시죠?

P : I have a stomachache.

위통이 있습니다.

N : Tell me about how you are feeling.

당신이 어떻게 느끼는 지 말해주세요.

P : I am suffering from indigestion and heartburn.

소화가 안 되고 속 쓰림을 느낍니다.

N : How long have you been having your discomfort?

얼마나 오랫동안 불편하셨나요?

P : It's been going on for a few weeks.

몇 주 정도 지속이 되었습니다.

N : Do you get worse after eating?

음식을 먹고 나면 더 악화가 되나요?

P : Yes.

예.

N : Have you ever had an upper gastrointestinal endoscopic
    examination?

상부 위장관 내시경을 받아 본 적이 있으십니까?

P : Yes. I had a regular medical check up last year.

네. 작년에 종합검진을 받았습니다.

Results were normal.

결과는 정상이었습니다.

N : OK. How old are you?

알겠습니다. 몇 살이시죠?

P : 38 years old.

38세입니다.

N : Really? You look much younger.

정말요? 나이에 비해 젊어 보이시네요.

P : Thank you.

고맙군요.

N : Are you married?

결혼은 하셨나요?

P : Yes.

네.

N : How many children do you have?

아이들은 명 몇이 있나요?

P : Two.

두 명입니다.

N : How old are they?

몇 살이지요?

P : My son is 9. My daughter is 7.

아들은 9살이고 딸은 7살입니다.

N : Do your children go to school?

아이들이 학교에 다니나요?

P : Yes. they do.

네. 그렇습니다.

N : Are your parents alive and in good health?

부모님들은 살아 계시고 건강하신가요?

P : Yes.

네.

N : What religion do you have?

종교가 무엇이지요?

P : Catholic.

카톨릭입니다.

N : What kind of work do you do?

어떤 일을 하시죠?

P : I work for a company.

회사에 다니고 있습니다.

My health broke down due to working day and night.

밤낮으로 일하다 보니 건강이 망가졌습니다.

N : Excessive working can undermine your health.

과도한 일은 당신의 건강을 서서히 무너뜨릴 수 있습니다.

P : How long is your work?

몇 시간 근무하세요?

N : We are with patients during 8 or12 hour shifts.

환자들과 8시간 또는 12시간 동안 같이합니다.

3. 환자의 과거 병력, 가족력 질문

Very Useful Expressions

1. I would like to review your past history prior to your admission.

   입원하기 전에 당신의 과거력을 물어보겠습니다.

2. Do you have any medical conditions?

   어떤 질환을 가지고 있나요?

3. Have you had any health problems recently?

   최근 당신의 건강에 문제가 되는 것들이 있었나요?

4. Have you ever had any medical attention?

   의학적인 주의를 받은 적이 있었나요?

5. Do you have any diseases, such as high blood pressure, diabetes, allergy, or hepatitis?

   고혈압이나 당뇨병, 알러지, 간염 같은 어떤 질환이 있습니까?

6. Could you tell me a little about your previous health?

   과거 건강상태에 대해 조금 말해 주실래요?

7. Do you have any other illnesses that you see a doctor for?

   의사에게 진료를 받은 다른 질병들이 있나요?

8. Have you ever had any serious illnesses or operations?

   과거에 아프거나 수술했던 적이 있나요?

9. Have you ever been in hospital for any reason?

어떤 이유로 입원한 적이 있나요?

10. What kind of operation have you had?

어떤 종류의 수술을 받으셨죠?

11. When was the date of operation?

수술 날짜가 언제죠?

12. Have you ever had an allergic reaction to any drug or injection?

어떤 약이나 주사에 부작용이 있었던 적이 있나요?

13. How about your health in the past?

당신의 과거 건강 상태는 어떠했습니까?

14. Is there anything else you'd like to tell me?

나에게 말하고 싶은 것이 있나요?

15. Do you have any family history of hypertension, diabetes or cancer?

고혈압이나 당뇨병, 암과 같은 가족력이 있나요?

환자의 과거력에 대해서 물어 볼 때는

I would like to review your past history. 로 시작하고

당신의 병력 전부를 듣고 싶습니다. 는

I'd like to take your full medical history. 라 말한다.

과거의 건강 상태를 물어 볼 때는

How about your health in the past?

Tell me about how your health been in the past.

Tell me about any serious illnesses you have had in the past.

최근의 건강 상태에 대해 물어 볼 때는

How has your health been?

어떤 의학적인 문제가 있는 지는

Do you have any medical conditions?

Have you ever had any medical problems?

Are you currently under the care of a doctor?

어떤 질병에 걸렸거나 수술을 받은 적이 있는 지는

Have you ever had any serious illnesses or operations?

수술 종류에 대해서는 What kind of operation have you had?

수술 날짜가 언제였는 지는

When was the date of operation?

지금도 치료받고 있나요? 는 Are you still being treated? 라 한다.

다른 의학적인 문제를 가지고 있나요? 는

Do you have any other medical problems?

당신을 괴롭히는 문제들이 있나요? 는

Has anything problems been bothering you?

환자에게 병력지에 기입해 주라는 부탁은

Would you please fill out this medical history form? 이다.

환자의 가족력에 대해서 물어 볼 때는

Are there any disease that you think run in your family?

Are there any illnesses that seem to run in your family?

현재 가족 중에 심하게 아픈 환자가 있는지는

Has anyone in your family been seriously ill?

혈압이나 당뇨, 암과 같은 가족력이 있는지는

Do you have family history of hypertension or diabetes or cancer? 등으로 물어본다.

Conversation

N : Good afternoon. I'll be one of the nurses taking care of you here.

안녕하세요. 저는 이곳에서 당신을 돌보아 줄 간호사 중 한 명입니다.

P : Nice to meet you.

반갑습니다.

N : I've been a nurse for 5 years now.

지금 5년째 간호사로 일하고 있습니다.

I see that you are here for knee arthroscopy.

보니까 이곳에 무릎 관절경술을 받으러 오신 것 같군요.

P : Yes.

네.

N : I have just got a few questions to ask you.

당신에게 몇 가지 물어볼 것들이 있습니다.

It won't take long. Is that OK?

오래 걸리지는 않을 것입니다. 괜찮겠어요?

P : OK.

알겠습니다.

N : When did your symptom seem to begin?

증상이 언제부터 시작되었던 것 같으시나요?

P : About 5 months ago, I started feeling pain on my right knee.

5달 전 우측 무릎에 통증이 시작되었습니다.

2 weeks ago, I helped move some heavy furniture.

2주 전 무거운 가구를 옮기는 것을 도와주었죠.

Pain got much worse afterward.

그 후로 통증이 악화되었어요.

N : I'd like to review your past history.

당신의 과거력을 물어보겠습니다.

Do you have any disease like high blood pressure, diabetes or allergy?

고혈압, 당뇨, 알러지 같은 질환은 없으신가요?

P : No.

없습니다.

N : Is there anything in your past history, such as hepatitis or tuberculosis?

과거에 간염이나 결핵 같은 질환은 없었나요?

P : No.

없습니다.

N : Have you ever had any serious illnesses or operations?

과거에 아프거나 수술했던 적이 있나요?

P : Last year I was hospitalized.

작년에 입원을 했었습니다.

N : Do you remember what the diagnosis was?

진단이 무엇이었는지 기억하십니까?

P : Acute gastric ulcer.

급성 위궤양이었습니다.

N : When were you hospitalized?

언제 입원하셨죠?

P : In early September, for about one week.

9월 초에, 약 일주일간입니다.

N : Are you cured at the moment?

지금은 다 치료가 되었나요?

P : Yes. I was completely healed.

네. 완전히 다 낳았습니다.

N : Are you afraid of operation?

수술이 두려우신가요?

P : Not really.

그렇지는 않아요?

N : Will someone from your family be here with you?

가족들 중 누군가가 당신과 함께 있으실거죠?

P : Yes.

네.

N : OK. Would you please fill out this medical history form?

알겠습니다. 이 과거 병력 양식에 기입을 해주실래요?

4. 입원환자의 신체 정보 질문

Very Useful Expressions

1. What's your height?

   How tall are you?

   Do you know your height?

   키가 얼마나 되시죠?

2. Would you please take off your shoes

   and stand on the height measuring machine?

   신발을 벗고 키 재는 기구에 서주실래요?

3. What's your weight?

   How much do you weigh?

   Do you know your weight?

   체중이 얼마이시죠?

4. Would you please step on the scale?

   체중계에 올라가 주실래요?

5. Please, step on the height weight measuring machine.

   키, 체중 측정기에 올라가 서 주실래요?

6. You may step down.

   내려 오셔도 됩니다.

7. Do you put on weight recently?

   최근에 살이 쪘나요?

8. Do you lose weight recently?

최근에 살이 빠졌나요?

9. Have you lost or gained weight recently?

최근에 체중이 불거나 줄어든 적이 있나요?

10. Please read this form and fill it out.

이 양식을 읽어보시고 기입을 해주실래요?

키가 얼마인지 물어 볼 때는

Can you tell me your height? How tall are you?

What's your height? Do you know your height?

체중이 얼마인지 물어 볼 때는

Can you tell me your weight? How much do you weigh?

Tell me about your present weight.

최근에 체중이 불거나 줄어든 적이 있는지는

Have you lost or gained weight recently?

체중의 변화가 있는 지는

Is there any change in your weight?

Do you have any recent weight change?로 물어본다.

체중계나 키 측정기 위로 올라가주시라는 표현은

Can you stand on the scales, please?

Would you please step on the scale?

Please, step on the height weight measuring machine.

등을 사용한다.

Conversation

N : Good morning. Have a seat.

안녕하세요. 자리에 앉으세요.

What brought you to this hospital?

어디가 불편해 이 병원에 오셨죠?

P : I have got a bad cough.

기침이 심합니다.

N : How long have you had this symptom?

증상이 얼마나 오래되었죠?

P : About a couple of weeks.

약 2주일 되었습니다.

N : Do you produce any phlegm when coughing?

기침을 할 때 가래가 나오나요?

P : Sometimes, but it's usually pretty dry.

가끔요. 하지만 대부분 마른 기침을 합니다.

N : Do you smoke?

담배를 피우시나요?

P : Yes, a few cigarettes a day.

하루에 몇 개 피웁니다.

Fewer than 10.

10개 이하입니다.

N : Do you have a fever?

열이 나시나요?

P : I don't seem to have a fever.

열은 없는 것 같습니다.

N : Have you seen another doctor?

다른 의사에게 진료 받은 적이 있나요?

P : No.

아닙니다.

N : I'd like to review your history.

당신의 과거력을 알고 싶군요.

How has your health been in the past?

당신의 과거 건강 상태는 어떠했습니까?

Have you ever had any serious illnesses or operations in

the past?

과거에 크게 아픈 적이나 수술을 받은 적이 있습니까?

P : I had an appendectomy 3 years ago.

3년 전에 충수돌기 절제술을 받았습니다.

N : Do you have any history of high blood pressure, diabetes,

allergy or any other disease?

고혈압, 당뇨병, 알러지 또는 어떤 다른 질환을 가진 적이 있습니까?

P : No.

없습니다.

N : How tall are you?

키가 얼마나 되시죠?

P : 174.

174cm입니다.

N : How much do you weigh?

체중이 얼마이시죠?

P : I don't know. I didn't measure my weight recently.

모르겠습니다. 최근에 몸무게를 측정해보지 않았습니다.

N : How much did you weigh in the past year?

지난 1년 동안에는 체중이 얼마였죠?

P : About 76kg.

약 76kg입니다.

N : Would you please step on the scale?

체중계에 올라가 주실래요?

P : Yes.

네.

N : Oh. You weigh 71kg.

아 71kg이네요.

P : It has changed recently.

최근 체중이 변했군요.

N : You may step down.

내려 오셔도 됩니다.

Put on your shoes.

신발을 신으세요.

Would you please sit over there?

저기 앉으실래요?

Why has your weight changed, do you think?

왜 체중이 변했다고 생각을 하죠?

42

Do you become fatigued easily?

쉽고 피곤해지나요?

P : Yes. I am suffering from loss of appetite.

네. 요즘 식욕이 없습니다.

N : What is the most you have ever weighed?

가장 체중이 많이 나갔던 게 얼마이셨죠?

P : 80kg.

80kg입니다.

N : Do you exercise regularly?

규칙적으로 운동을 하십니까?

P : No.

아닙니다.

N : Have you ever had any medical attention to your problem?

당신의 증상에 대해 의학적인 주의를 받은 적이 있나요?

P : No.

없습니다.

N : I'll take your blood pressure

혈압을 측정해 보겠습니다.

Will you roll up your sleeve?

소매를 좀 올려주실래요?

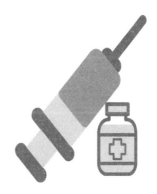

5. 활력징후(혈압, 맥박, 체온) 측정

Very Useful Expressions

1. I'll check your vital signs.

   활력징후를 측정하겠습니다.

2. I am going to take your blood pressure, pulse
   and temperature.

   당신의 혈압과 맥박, 체온을 측정하겠습니다.

3. Let me take your blood pressure.

   혈압을 측정하겠습니다.

4. Would you please take off your jacket
   and roll up your sleeve?

   재킷을 벗고 소매를 올려 주실래요?

5. Would you please put your arm on the automatic
   blood pressure monitor?

   자동 혈압계에 팔을 올려 주실래요?

6. Fine. It's quite normal.

   정상이군요.

7. Your blood pressure is 140 over 90.

   혈압이 140에 90이군요.

8. Normal blood pressure is 120 over 80.

   정상 혈압은 120에 80입니다.

44

9. I'll take your pulse.

맥박을 측정하겠습니다.

10. You have a slow pulse. It's 46.

당신은 46회 서맥이군요.

11. You have a pulse of 64 and a BP of 125 over 80.

맥박이 64이고 혈압이 125에 80이군요.

12. I'll check your temperature.

체온을 측정해보겠습니다.

13. Temperature is normal.

체온이 정상입니다.

14. Temperature goes up. It's 39C.

체온이 39도로 올랐네요.

15. Your temperature has increased to 38C.

체온이 38도로 올랐네요.

16. Your respirations are slow at 12 breaths a minute.

당신의 호흡은 분당 12회로 느리군요.

혈압이나 맥박, 체온을 측정할 때는

Take, Check 동사를 주로 사용하는데,

혈압을 잴 때는

Let me check your blood pressure.

I'll take your blood pressure.

I want to check your blood pressure.

I am going to take your blood pressure. 등으로 표현한다.

맥박을 잴 때는 Let me take your pulse.

체온을 잴 때는 Let me check your temperature.

귀를 통해 체온을 측정할 때는

I'll check your temperature through your ear.

구강으로 체온을 측정하겠다는 표현은

I'll check your temperature by mouth.

체온계를 혀 아래에 물고 계시라는 표현은

Please hold the thermometer under your tongue.이다.

고혈압이 있는 지 물어볼 때는

Do you have high blood pressure?

전에 혈압이 높았던 적이 있는 지는

Has your blood pressure been high before? 라고 물어본다.

검사를 할 때 긴장하는 환자들에게

편하게 하라고 말할 수 있는 표현들은

Relax. Try to relax. Let yourself go loose. Take it easy. 이고,

검사가 다 끝났다는 표현은

We are done. We finished. We all finished.

All done. It's finished. It's done. 등이다.

Conversation

N : Can you tell me your problem?

무슨 문제가 있으시죠?

P : I've got a headache.

두통이 있습니다.

N : How long have you been suffering from headache?

두통을 얼마 동안 느끼셨죠?

P : These past few days.

요 며칠간입니다.

N : Are you having any other problems?

다른 증상은 없으시나요?

P : I'm feeling ill.

몸이 아픕니다.

N : Where does it hurt the most?

어디가 가장 아프죠?

P : I feel pain all over my body.

몸 전체가 아픕니다.

And I've also had a little bit of diarrhea.

그리고 약간의 설사를 합니다.

N : How about allergies?

알러지는 없으시나요?

Do you have any allergies?

알러지가 있으신가요?

P : Not that I'm aware of.

제가 알기로는 없습니다.

N : OK. I'll take your blood pressure.

알겠습니다. 혈압을 측정하겠습니다.

Can I have your arm?

팔 좀 주실래요?

Will you roll up your sleeve?

소매를 올려 주실래요?

P : OK.

알겠습니다.

N : Don't grip your hand and relax.

손을 쥐지 말고 푸세요.

I am going to place a cuff around your arm.

커프를 팔에 감을게요.

It will be a little tight.

약간 조이는 느낌이 드실 겁니다.

Has your blood pressure been high before?

전에 혈압이 높았던 적이 있었나요?

P : Not that I know of.

제가 알기로는 없습니다.

N : Your blood pressure is fine.

혈압은 정상이시군요.

Blood pressure is 120 over 80.

혈압이 120에 80입니다.

I'll take your pulse.

맥박을 측정하겠습니다.

It's OK.

괜찮군요.

P : I am feeling under the weather today.

오늘 몸이 안 좋습니다.

N : Do you have a fever?

열이 있나요?

I'll check your temperature through your ear.

귀를 통해 체온을 측정하겠습니다.

Your temperature goes up to 38 C.

체온이 38도까지 오르셨네요.

I just need to check a few things with you.

당신에게 체크해야 할 것들이 몇 가지 있습니다.

Please read this form and fill it out.

이 양식을 읽어보시고 기입을 해주세요.

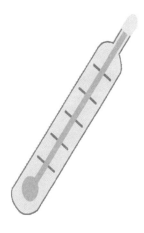

6. 먹고 있는 약에 대한 질문

Very Useful Expressions

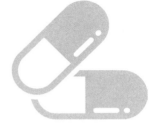

1. Are you taking any medication?
   어떤 약을 먹고 있나요?

2. What medications do you take?
   무슨 약을 먹고 있으시죠?

3. Why are you taking it?
   왜 약을 복용하고 계시죠?

4. How long have you been taking the medication?
   얼마나 오랫동안 약을 복용하고 있으셨죠?

5. When do you take it?
   언제 약을 복용하시죠?

6. Did you take your medicine today?
   오늘 약을 드셨나요?

7. Are you allergic to any medicines?
   어떤 약에 알러지가 있나요?

현재 먹고 있는 약이 있는 지 물어보려면

Are you having any medications you are currently taking?

Are you on any medication?

Are you currently taking any medicines?

Do you take any medication? 등으로 표현할 수 있다.

어떤 약을 복용하고 있는 지는

What medications do you take?

What medications are you currently taking?

왜 약을 복용하고 있는 지는

Why are you taking it?

What are you taking that for?

얼마나 복용하고 있는 지는

How much are you taking?

얼마나 오래 약을 복용하고 있는 지는

How long have you been taking the medication?

얼마나 자주 복용하는 지는

How often do you take the medication?

언제 약을 복용하는 지는

When do you take it? 로 물어 본다.

약의 복용에 대한 약자는

q.d (quaque die)-every day, b.i.d (bis in die)-twice a day,

t.i.d (ter in die)-three times a day, q.i.d (quater in die)-four

times a day, q.h (quaque hora)-every hour 등이다.

Conversation

N : Do you take pain-killers sometimes?

진통제를 가끔씩 드시나요?

P : No.

아뇨.

N : Are you taking any medication?

어떤 약을 먹고 있나요?

P : Yes.

네.

N : What medications are you currently taking?

지금 어떤 약을 먹고 계시죠?

P : Hypertension medicines.

고혈압 약입니다.

N : How long have you been taking it?

얼마나 오랫동안 복용하셨죠?

P : About 5 years.

약 5년입니다.

N : Did you take it today?

오늘도 약을 드셨나요?

P : Yes.

네.

N : I am going to take your blood pressure.

혈압을 측정하겠습니다.

Can I have your arm?

팔 좀 주실래요?

Your blood pressure is 130 over 85.

혈압이 130에 85입니다.

Are you married?

결혼은 했나요?

P : Yes.

예.

N : Could you tell me a little bit about your family?

당신의 가족에 대해서 말씀 좀 해주실래요?

P : What would you like to know?

무엇을 알고 싶으시죠?

N : How long have you been married?

결혼한 지 얼마나 오래 되었지요?

P : 5 years.

5년 되었습니다.

N : How many people are there in your family?

가족이 모두 몇 명이지요?

P : Three.

3 명입니다.

N : Do you have only one child?

애가 한 명밖에 없나요?

P : Yes. one girl.

예. 딸 하나입니다.

N : How old is she?

아이가 몇 살이지요?

P : 3 years old.

3살입니다.

N : What about your bowel movements?

배변 습관은 어떤가요?

P : I go once a day, in the morning.

아침에 한 번씩 갑니다.

N : Have you lost or gained weight recently?

최근에 체중에 어떤 변화가 있었습니까?

P : I have lost weight recently.

최근에 몸무게가 줄었습니다.

N : What did you weigh 6 months ago?

6달 전에는 몸무게가 얼마였죠?

P : Sixty-nine kilogram.

69kg이었습니다.

N : And now?

지금은 얼마죠?

P : Sixty kilogram.

60kg입니다.

N: OK. Can you describe your smoking and drinking habits?

알겠습니다. 담배나 음주습관에 대해 말해주실래요?

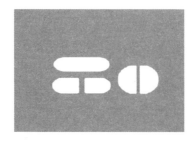

7. 술과 담배에 대한 질문

Very Useful Expressions

1. I'd like to check your smoking and drinking habits.
   당신의 흡연과 음주 습관에 대해 알고 싶습니다.

2. Do you drink?
   술을 드시나요?

3. Are you a heavy drinker?
   술을 많이 마시나요?

4. How much alcohol do you drink per week?
   일주일에 얼마만큼 술을 드시죠?

5. Do you have any gastric discomfort or liver problem?
   위 불편감이나 간 문제가 있지는 않나요?

6. Do you smoke?
   담배를 피우나요?

7. How much do you smoke?
   담배를 얼마나 피우시죠?

8. One pack a day? More than one pack a day? Two packs?
   하루 한 갑인가요? 하루 한 갑 이상인가요? 두 갑?

9. No more than a half a pack a day?
   하루에 반 갑 이하입니까?

10. How many years have you smoked?

몇 년 동안 피우셨나요?

11. Do you cough up phlegm?

가래가 나오나요?

12. Do you have any difficulty with your breathing?

숨을 쉬는데 불편하지는 않나요?

술을 마시는지 물어볼 때는

Do you drink?

술을 많이 마시는 지 물어볼 경우엔

Are you a heavy drinker?

술을 자주 마시는지는

Do you drink steadily? How often do you drink?

얼마나 오랫동안 술을 드셨는지는 For how long?

술을 얼마나 마시는지는 How much do you drink? 로 표현한다.

환자에게 담배를 피우고 있는지 질문을 할 때는

Do you smoke?

얼마나 피는지는 How much do you smoke?

How many cigarettes do you smoke a day?

언제부터 피웠는지는

When did you start smoking?

How many years have you been smoked?

등으로 물어본다.

Conversation

N : Do you smoke?

담배를 피우나요?

P : Yes.

네.

N : How many cigarettes do you smoke a day?

하루에 담배를 몇 개를 피우시죠?

P : I smoke a pack a day.

하루 한 갑을 피웁니다.

N : Is that as much as you have always smoked?

그 양이 당신이 항상 피우는 양입니까?

P : Sometimes more, sometimes less.

때론 많이 피기도 하고 때론 적게 핍니다.

N : When did you start smoking?

언제 흡연을 시작하셨죠?

P : 20 years old.

20살부터입니다.

N : Do you drink?

술을 마시나요?

P : Yes.

네.

N : Are you a heavy drinker?

술을 많이 마시나요?

P : I am a moderate drinker.

적당히 마십니다.

N : Do you drink every day?

매일 술을 마시나요?

P : No. a couple of times a week.

아닙니다. 일주일에 2번 정도입니다.

N : How much do you drink on average?

보통 얼마나 마시죠?

P : Half a bottle of whiskey.

위스키 반 병 정도입니다.

N : Have you ever had a drinking problem?

음주 때문에 문제가 된 적이 있나요?

P : No.

아닙니다.

N : What is your work?

무슨 일을 하시죠?

P : I am out of work at present.

지금은 실직상태입니다.

N : How long have you been out of work?

직업이 없는 지 얼마나 되셨죠?

P : 2 years.

2 년 되었습니다.

N : Please describe your symptoms.

증상을 말해 주실래요?

P : Maybe a little bit trouble with my wind.

아무래도 숨을 쉬는데 문제가 있는 것 같습니다.

I don't breathe as well as I used to.

평상시처럼 숨을 쉴 수가 없습니다.

It's probably just the cigarettes.

아마도 담배 때문이겠지요.

N : Are your parents still alive?

당신의 부모님은 모두 살아 계신가요?

P : My mother is living.

어머니는 살아계십니다.

But my father passed away when he was 62.

하지만 아버지는 62세에 돌아가셨습니다.

N : What did he pass away from?

왜 돌아가셨지요?

P : Colon cancer.

대장암으로 돌아가셨습니다.

N : How about your mother?

어머니는 어떠신가요?

P : She is in good health.

그녀는 건강하십니다.

N : OK. Fill out this paper and return it.

알겠습니다. 이 설문지를 채우시고 돌려주세요.

8. 대변과 소변에 관한 질문

Very Useful Expressions

1. How about your bowel movements?
   대변을 보는 것은 어떻습니까?

2. Do you have any trouble having a bowel movement?
   대변을 보는데 무슨 문제가 있습니까?

3. Do you have bowel movements today?
   오늘 대변을 보았습니까?

4. How many bowel movements do you have today?
   오늘 대변을 몇 번 보았습니까?

5. How about your urination?
   소변을 보는 것은 어떻습니까?

6. Do you have any problems passing water?
   소변을 보는데 무슨 문제가 있습니까?

7. Any problems with your waterworks?
   소변을 보는 것은 문제가 없나요?

8. Is everything all right?
   Bowel movements and urination?
   대변이나 소변을 보는 것이 모두 괜찮습니까?

대변을 본다는 Bowel Movement,

소변은 Pass Water, Take a leak, Urination, Water Works 란

단어들을 지역에 따라 다르게 사용하는데,

대변 습관에 대해서 물어 볼 때는

How are the bowel movements?

What about your bowel movements? Are the bowels all right?

Do you have any trouble having bowel movements?

소변을 보는 것이 어떤 지는

How about your urination? How is the water?

How are the water works?

Do you have any problems passing water?

Do you have any problems taking a leak?

Any problems with your waterworks? 라고 물어본다.

설사를 했는지 물어볼 때는

Do you have diarrhea?

Do you have soft stool? Do you have watery stool?

대변에 피가 보이는지는

Is there blood in the stools? 등으로 물어본다.

소변을 보기 어려운지는

Do you have any difficulty with urination?

소변에 피가 보이는지는 Is there bloody urine?

소변이 찔끔거리는지는

Do you have urine dribbling? 등으로 물어본다.

Conversation

N : Have you recently had an endoscopy or an ultrasound scan
of your abdomen?

최근에 내시경이나 복부 초음파 검사를 받았습니까?

P : Yes and the results were all right.

네. 결과는 정상이었습니다.

But I have had chronic belching.

하지만 자주 트림이 나옵니다.

N : How about your bowel movements?

대변을 보는 것은 어떻습니까?

Do you have any black bowel movements?

검은색 변을 보지는 않습니까?

P : No, my stool is dark brown.

아뇨, 대변 색깔은 짙은 갈색입니다.

N : What does the stool look like?

대변 모양은 어떻죠?

Watery stools? Hard stools?

설사인가요? 된 변인가요?

P : Soft stools.

묽은 변입니다.

N : Any sign of blood?

출혈은 안보이나요?

P : No.

아닙니다.

N : Do you have any problems passing water?

소변을 보는 것은 문제가 없나요?

P : No trouble.

아무 문제가 없습니다.

N : Do you have any other problem?

다른 문제는 없나요?

P : I am diabetic.

당뇨병이 있습니다.

N : Are you taking any tablet or insulin?

약을 먹거나 인슐린을 맞고 있나요?

P : I am taking insulin for my diabetes.

당뇨병 치료를 위해 인슐린을 맞고 있습니다.

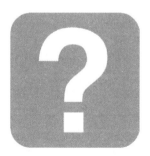

9. 전원을 오거나 전원이 필요한 경우

Very Useful Expressions

1. Which hospital were you staying at?
   어느 병원에 입원을 하였었나요?

2. Would you give me a doctor's note?
   의사소견서를 저에게 주실래요?

3. Do you bring any relevant X-rays or test results?
   관련되는 x-ray 필름이나 결과지들을 가져 오셨나요?

4. Do you bring your medication?
   당신의 약들은 가져 왔나요?

5. Please bring your medicines and prescription.
   당신의 약이나 처방전을 병원으로 가져와 주세요.

6. We'd like to discuss regarding your conditions.
   당신의 상태에 대해 상의할 것이 있습니다.

7. We are concerned about the progress of the disease.
   병의 진행 상황에 대해 점점 걱정이 됩니다.

8. I am afraid your illness is more serious than
   first we thought.
   당신의 병이 처음 생각한 것 보다 더 심각합니다.

9. Our hospital cannot provide the treatment you need.
   우리 병원에서는 당신에게 필요한 치료를 하지 못 합니다.

10. You may be transferred to another hospital that can treat
   you.

   당신을 치료할 수 있는 다른 병원으로 전원이 필요할지 모릅니다.

11. If transfer is needed, doctor will discuss this with you
   and your family.

   전원이 필요하면 선생님이 당신과 가족들에게 상의할 것입니다.

의사 소견서는 Doctor's Note,

전원소견서는 Transfer note

또는 Patient Clinical Handover record

임상 검사 결과는 Laboratory Test Results 라고 하며,

의사 소견서와 결과지를 가지고 왔는지 물어볼 때는

Do you bring a Doctor's note and laboratory test results?

Do you have transfer note of other hospital?

등으로 표현한다.

안타깝게도 결과가 좋지 않다는 표현은

I am afraid results are not as good as expected.

병이 심각하다고 할 경우에는

I am afraid your disease is serious.

Your disease is unfortunately in a bad way.

Your illness is more serious than we first thought.

증상이 치료에 반응이 없다는 표현은

Your symptom hasn't responded to treatment.

적절한 치료를 하지 않으면 심각해 질 수 있다는 표현은

Without proper treatment, this can lead to complications.

당신을 치료 할 수 있는 대학 병원으로 전원이 필요합니다. 는

You need to be transferred to university hospital

that can treat you. 로 표현한다.

Conversation

N : Would you describe your symptom?

당신의 증상을 설명 해 주실래요?

P : My knee pain starts to get better with a period of inactivity,

but as soon as I do something like walk, pain is back.

무릎 통증이 활동을 안 할 때는 괜찮은데, 걷거나 조금만 활동을 해도

통증이 생깁니다.

Pain is felt while walking or standing for more than a few

minutes.

몇 분만 걷거나 서 있어도 통증을 느낍니다.

N : Have you seen another doctor recently?

최근에 다른 의사 선생님에게 진료를 받으셨나요?

P : Yes. I saw a doctor about a week ago.

네. 약 일주일전 의사선생님에게 진료를 받았었습니다.

Actually I had been hospitalized A hospital.

사실 A병원에 입원하였었습니다.

Doctor wanted me to go though surgery.

의사 선생님이 수술을 원하시더군요.

But I was not sure he was diagnosing my problem right.

하지만 그가 제 문제를 정확히 진단했는지 확신이 안 들었습니다.

N : Do you have doctor's note?

의사소견서는 가지고 계시나요?

P : Yes. Here it is.

네. 여기 있습니다.

N : Do you bring any relevant X-ray films or test results?

관련되는 x-ray 필름이나 결과지들을 가져 오셨나요?

P : No. I brought just doctor's note.

아뇨. 의사소견서만 가져왔습니다.

N : Are you currently taking any medicines?

지금 어떤 약들을 복용하시고 있나요?

P : I am taking hypertension medicine.

고혈압 약을 복용하고 있습니다.

N : Do you bring your medicine?

당신의 약들은 가져 왔나요?

P : I am afraid. I left them at home.

집에 약들을 두고 온 것 같습니다.

N : Did you come with your family?

가족들과 함께 오셨나요?

P : Yes.

네.

N : You need to send your family there.

가족을 집으로 보내셔야 할 것 같습니다.

Please bring your medicines and prescription to the hospital.

당신의 약이나 처방전을 병원으로 가져와 주세요.

P : OK.

알겠습니다.

N : Could you put your signature here?

이곳에 사인해 주실래요?

P : OK.

알겠습니다.

N : Will you need help with your luggage?

짐 옮기는데 도움이 필요하세요?

P : No, thank you.

아닙니다. 감사합니다.

N : Let me carry your luggage.

제가 짐을 들어 드릴께요.

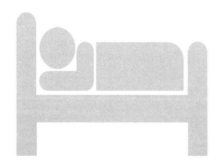

10. 입원에 대한 기본적인 설명들

Very Useful Expressions

1. Personal items, like a gown, towel and slippers will be provided by the hospital.
   병원 가운이나 수건, 슬리퍼는 병원에서 줄 것입니다.

2. You need to prepare personal toiletries.
   개인적인 세면도구는 준비를 하셔야 합니다.

3. You can buy daily necessaries at convenience store.
   생활용품들을 매점에서 살 수 있습니다.

4. Please don't bring anything of value into the hospital.
   값이 나가는 물건들은 병원에 가져오시면 안 됩니다.

5. You should give your valuables to your family.
   귀중품은 가족들에게 맡기십시오.

6. Please don't bring in electrical items except notebook.
   노트북을 제외한 전자제품은 가져오시면 안 됩니다.

7. You don't have to use electric heater or cooking pot.
   전기히터나 전기솥을 사용하시면 안 됩니다.

8. Please remove jewelry, makeup and nail polish before your admission.
   입원하기 전 귀금속, 화장, 손톱을 정리하시기 바랍니다.

9. Wi-Fi is available in all hospital areas.
   와이파이는 병원 전 지역에서 사용하실 수 있습니다.

10. Normal visiting hours are from 10 am to 8 pm.
    정상적인 병문안 시간은 오전 10시부터 오후 8시입니다.

11. If you feel any discomfort, please let us know.
    어디 불편한 곳이 있으면 저희들에게 알려주세요.

12. Please change into the hospital gown.
    환자복으로 갈아 입어주세요.

13. I'll show you how to use the emergency call.
    응급벨을 어떻게 사용하는 지 알려드리겠습니다.

14. You are not supposed to go out of the hospital.
    병원 밖으로 외출하시면 안 됩니다.

입원환자에게 세면도구와 같은
개인적인 생활 물품들을 준비해야 한다는
You need to prepare personal toiletries.
화장실에는 일회용 세면도구들이 없습니다. 는
Bathrooms don't include complimentary toiletries.
병원에서는 지갑을 안전하게 보관하십시오. 는
Please keep your wallet safely in the hospital.
항상 주머니에 지갑을 가지고 계시는 것이 좋을 것입니다. 는
You'd better always keep your wallet in your pocket.
만약 긴급한 일이 있으면 비상벨을 눌러주세요. 는
If there is anything urgent, press the emergency bell. 이다.

Conversation

P : Do I have to prepare slippers and toiletries personally?

슬리퍼나 세면도구는 스스로 준비를 해야 하나요?

N : Yes. You can buy daily necessaries at convenience store.

네. 생활용품들은 매점에서 사실 수 있습니다.

P : Can I use Wi-Fi?

와이파이는 사용할 수 있나요?

N : Yes. All patients can log on with this ID and password without

any limits during your stay.

네. 이 ID와 비밀번호로 병원에서 제약 없이 사용할 수 있습니다.

P : Can I use my cell phone?

제 핸드폰을 사용해도 되죠?

N : Yes. The use of mobile phones is permitted in the ward.

네. 핸드폰 사용은 병동에서 허용되어 있습니다.

And if necessary, a hospital telephone is available at the

nurse station.

그리고 필요하다면 병원 전화도 간호사실에서 사용할 수 있습니다.

P : What time are visiting hours at this hospital?

이 병원의 병문안 시간이 몇 시이죠?

N : Visiting hours are from 11 am to 2 pm, from 5pm to 8pm.

방문시간은 오전11시−오후 2시, 오후 5시−저녁 8시까지 입니다.

Please speak to the nursing staff about visiting outside of

these hours.

이 시간 이후에는 간호사들에게 말씀을 해주세요.

We ask you be mindful of other patient's comfort when visitors come in to see you.

방문객들이 당신을 보러 올 때, 다른 환자들에게 방해가 되지 않게 해주시기를 부탁드립니다.

P : OK.

알겠습니다.

N : If you require a special diet, please inform us as soon as possible.

만약 특별식이 필요하면 저희들에게 빨리 알려주세요.

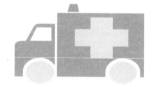

11. 회진(라운딩)중 필요한 표현들

Very Useful Expressions

1. How do you feel this morning?

오늘 아침은 어떠세요?

2. Do you feel much better?

더 나아지셨나요?

3. You are looking much better.

더 좋아진 것 같군요.

4. Did you sleep well last night?

어젯밤에는 잘 주무셨어요?

5. Did you get any sleep?

잠 좀 주무셨어요?

6. Weren't you cold last night?

지난 밤 춥지 않으셨어요?

7. Are you warm enough? Are you cold?

따뜻하셨나요? 추우셨나요?

8. Do you feel any discomfort?

어디 불편한 것은 없으세요?

9. Don't you feel well? You look so down.

어디 안 좋으세요? 보기에 안 좋으신 것 같군요.

10. Do you have any pain? Are you all right?

어디가 아프세요? 괜찮으신가요?

11. You don't look so good.

좋아 보이지 않군요.

12. Get some sleep.

잠 좀 주무세요.

13. Did you eat your meal?

아침식사는 드셨나요?

14. What's your appetite like?

식욕은 어떠세요?

15. You don't seem to have much appetite.

식욕이 없으신가 보군요.

16. You don't seem to get well yet.

아직 회복이 되지 않으신 것 같군요.

17. You will feel better soon.

곧 좋아지실 겁니다.

18. I hope you feel better soon.

곧 좋아지시길 바랍니다.

19. If you have difficulty washing your face and brushing
teeth, you can ask for help.

세수나 양치질이 어려우면 도움을 청하십시오.

20. If you can't go to the bathroom, feel free to ask for help.

화장실 가기 힘이 드시면 주저 없이 도움을 청하십시오.

21. Have your family members or friends visited you?

가족들이나 친구들이 병문안 왔었나요?

22. Sometimes open the windows and let fresh air in.

간혹 창문을 열고 환기를 시키십시오.

23. It's good to see you're healing.

당신이 나아가고 있는 것을 보니 좋군요.

24. You will be discharged soon.

곧 퇴원하게 될 것입니다.

회진 중 오늘은 조금 어떠냐는 표현은

How are you feeling today?

전보다 좋아 보인다는 말은 You look better than before.

기분이 좋은 것 같다는 표현은

You seem to be in a good mood.

기분이 좋지 않으신 것 같다는

You seem to be not in good condition.

잠을 잘 주무셨나요? 는 Did you sleep well?

잠을 잘 못 주무신 것 같군요. It looks like you didn't sleep well.

잠을 충분히 못 잔 이유가 있나요? 는

Is there any reason why you can't get enough sleep?

잠을 자지 못할 정도로 불편했나요? 는

Didn't you get comfortable enough to stay asleep? 로,

그리고 불편한 점이 있으면 알려주세요. 는

If you feel any discomfort, just let us know. 로 표현한다.

75

Conversation

N : Hi, there. Did you sleep well last night?

안녕하세요. 어젯밤 잘 주무셨어요?

P : I am not used to sleep in an unfamiliar place.

낯선 곳에서 자는 것이 익숙하지가 않습니다.

I slept fitfully.

자다 깨다 했습니다.

N : At the beginning, everyone feels uncomfortable in hospital.

처음에는 누구나 다 병원생활에 적응이 안 됩니다.

But don't worry.

You can gradually adapt to hospital environments.

하지만 걱정 마세요. 점점 더 병원 환경에 적응이 되실 것입니다.

Make yourself at home.

맘 편히 지내십시오.

How is your appetite?

식욕은 어떠세요?

P : Not bad.

괜찮아요.

N : Did you feel any pain through the night?

밤에 통증은 없으셨나요?

P : It was bearable.

견딜만 했습니다.

N : That's a relief.

다행이네요.

But you look so down.

하지만 어디 좋지 않으신 것 같네요.

Do you have any new symptoms?

새로운 증상 같은 것은 없나요?

P : No, but I am not in a good condition.

아니요. 그런데 상태가 좋지는 않습니다.

When will my doctor be here?

제 담당 선생님은 언제 오시죠?

N : Your doctor will soon come round to see you.

담당선생님이 곧 회진하러 오실 것입니다.

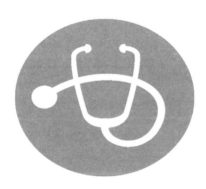

12. 환자 상태에 대한 질문과 답변들

Very Useful Expressions

1. How do you feel today?

   오늘은 어떠세요?

2. Do you have any pain?

   통증이 있으세요?

3. How bad is your pain?

   통증이 얼마나 심하시죠?

4. Is the pain tolerable?

   통증은 참을 만 하나요?

5. Is there any change in your symptom?

   증상의 변화가 있으신가요?

6. Has everything been OK with you?

   다 괜찮으신가요?

7. Do you have any problems moving your bowels?

   대변보는 것에 문제는 없나요?

8. Do you have any problems taking a leak?

   소변보는 것에 문제는 없나요?

9. Did you break wind (fart)?

   방귀를 뀌셨나요?

10. Are you having trouble breathing?

숨을 쉬기 힘이 드시나요?

11. Do you get any pain in your chest?

가슴이 아픕니까?

12. Do you have any abdominal discomfort?

복부 불편감이 있으신가요?

13. Do you feel nausea or vomiting?

오심이나 구토를 느끼나요?

14. We got your test results.

검사 결과가 나왔습니다.

15. All looks fine.

모든 것이 좋은 것 같습니다.

16. There doesn't seem to be anything wrong with you.

당신에게는 특별한 이상이 없는 것 같군요.

17. Your blood and urine tests are normal.

혈액과 소변 검사는 정상입니다.

18. We don't think it's anything serious.

심각한 것은 아니라고 생각합니다.

19. Doctor will explain about your results in detail.

의사 선생님이 결과들을 자세히 설명을 해 주실 것입니다.

20. Do you feel uncomfortable?

어디 불편하신가요?

21. Are you gonna throw up?

토할 것 같나요?

22. We'll get you something as soon as we can.

가능한 빨리 조치해 주겠습니다.

23. The doctor will be here soon.

의사 선생님이 곧 오실 것입니다.

지금은 어떠세요? 는

How are you feeling at the moment?

오늘은 어떠세요? 는

How are you feeling today? 또는 How do you feel today?

오늘 통증이 어떤지는 How is your pain feeling today?

오늘 증상이 더 좋아졌는지는 Do you feel much better today?

또는 Are you feeling any better today? 로 물어 본다.

그리고 환자가 결과에 대해 궁금해 할 때는,

X-ray 와 혈액 검사 결과가 나왔습니다.

Your X-rays and test results are back.

혈액과 소변 검사가 정상입니다.

Your blood and urine tests are normal.

모든 게 정상 인 것 같습니다. All seems to appear normal.

걱정할 이유가 없습니다. There is no reason to worry.

심각한 것이 아닙니다. It's nothing serious.

의사 선생님이 결과를 자세히 설명을 해 주실 것입니다.

Doctor will explain about your results in detail. 로 말한다.

Conversation

N : Blood pressure was 150 over 90 early in the morning.

이른 아침 혈압이 150에 90이었습니다.

It was a little higher than it should be.

정상 수치보다는 약간 높더군요.

Has your blood pressure been high before?

전에 혈압이 높았던 적이 있었나요?

P : Not that I know of.

제가 알기로는 없습니다.

N : I'd like to check again.

다시 한 번 확인하고 싶군요.

Can I have your arm?

팔 좀 주실래요?

Will you tuck up your sleeve?

소매를 올려 주시겠어요?

P : OK.

알겠습니다.

N : Your blood pressure is 125 over 80.

혈압이 125에 80입니다.

You have a normal blood pressure at the moment.

지금은 정상 혈압이시네요.

It may be a temporary condition.

아마도 일시적인 현상 같습니다.

How do you feel today?

오늘은 좀 어떠세요?

Do you feel uncomfortable?

어디 불편하신가요?

P : I am feeling under the weather.

몸이 안 좋습니다.

Do I have a fever?

제가 열이 있나요?

N : I am not sure.

잘 모르겠습니다.

Let me take your temperature.

체온을 재어보겠습니다.

Your temperature goes up to 38 C.

체온이 38도까지 오르셨네요.

I will report your fever to a doctor.

열이 난다고 의사선생님에게 알리겠습니다.

Doctor will prescribe a fever reducer a little while later.

의사선생님이 잠시 후 해열제를 처방해 줄 것입니다.

P : OK. Thank you.

알겠습니다. 감사합니다.

13. 주사를 놓을 때

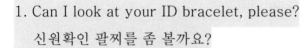

Very Useful Expressions

1. Can I look at your ID bracelet, please?

   신원확인 팔찌를 좀 볼까요?

2. I'll start the intravenous(IV) injection.

   정맥 주사를 놓겠습니다.

3. It'll sting a little.

   약간 따끔합니다.

4. The doctor wants to take some blood tests.

   의사 선생님이 혈액 검사를 원하십니다.

5. I'll take a sample of blood.

   혈액 샘플을 빼겠습니다.

6. It won't be painful (sore).

   아프지 않을 것입니다.

7. Can you roll up your sleeve?

   소매를 올려 줄래요?

8. Can you put your arm out straight?

   팔을 쭉 펴주실래요?

9. Can you hold out your hand?

   손을 내밀어 주실래요?

10. Can you turn your head to other side for me, please?

저를 위해 머리를 다른 쪽으로 돌려주실래요?

11. Please, grip your hand.

손을 쥐어주세요.

12. You haven't get a good vein anywhere.

어느 곳에도 괜찮은 정맥이 없군요.

13. It will hurt a bit.

약간 아플 것입니다.

14. I got it.

됐습니다.

15. Relax your fist.

주먹을 푸세요.

16. Can you bend your arm, please?

팔을 구부려 주실래요?

17. We are finished now.

끝났습니다.

18. You could be nauseous for a while after your injection.

주사 후 약간 메스꺼울 수 있습니다.

19. I'll give you the intramuscular(IM) injection.

근육 주사를 놓겠습니다.

20. Lie on your stomach. (Lie on your front.)

엎드리세요.

21. Could you turn on your left side?

왼쪽으로 돌아서 누우실래요?

22. Could you slip your trousers down?

바지를 아래로 내려 주실래요?

23. Please lower your pants and underwear.

바지와 속옷을 내려 주세요.

24. During an intramuscular injection, make sure the muscle
is relaxed.

근육 주사를 놓는 동안 근육의 긴장을 푸세요.

25. If your muscle is tight, it will likely hurt more.

근육이 긴장되면 더 아플 것입니다.

26. If the site swells or turns red, just let us know.

만약 주사 부위가 붓거나 붉어지면 알려주세요.

27. Use an ice pack on the injection site.

주사 맞은 자리에 얼음찜질을 하세요.

28. Let's take the IV out.

정맥 주사를 뺄게요.

혈액 채취가 필요합니다. 는

We need to do a blood sampling.

약간의 혈액을 빼겠습니다. 는

I am going to draw some blood.

정맥주사를 놓겠습니다.

I'll give you an IV injection.

주먹을 꼭 쥐어 주세요. Clench your fist.

정맥이 어디에도 없군요.

You haven't get a vein anywhere.

중심 정맥이 필요할 것 같군요.

You are going to need a central line.

만약 이상한 느낌이 들면 알려주세요.

If you feel any discomfort, just let me know.

If any of abnormal symptoms occur, just call me. 이다.

3방향 정맥주사 라인을 유지한다는 표현은

We need to keep the three-way stopcock on the IV line.

엉덩이에 주사를 놓겠습니다.

I will give you an injection in your buttocks.

주사의 흔한 부작용은 통증과 국소 자극입니다.

Common side effects of injections include

pain and local irritation.

주사 부위를 마사지하거나 문질러 주세요.

Massage and rub the injection site.

이것이 약물을 퍼지게 하거나 근육을 느슨하게 해줍니다. 는

This will help disperse the medication and loosen the muscle.

이다.

Conversation

N : Did you sleep well?

잘 주무셨어요?

P : I haven't slept well the past few days.

며칠간 잠을 잘 못 잤습니다.

N : I am sorry to hear that.

안 되었군요.

Try to get some sleep in the morning.

아침에 잠 좀 주무세요.

P : OK.

알겠습니다.

N : I need to draw some blood.

약간의 혈액을 빼겠습니다.

And I'll give you an IV injection.

그리고 정맥주사를 놓겠습니다.

Grip your hand.

주먹을 꼭 쥐어 주세요.

You have been sustained intravenously for so long that your

arm veins are useless for IV.

너무 오랫동안 주사를 맞아 와서 당신 팔의 정맥에 주사를 못 놓겠군요.

I'd like to use your leg veins.

당신의 다리에 있는 정맥을 이용하겠습니다.

P : It hurts.

아프군요.

N : Oh! I missed the vein.

이런 정맥으로 안 들어갔군요.

I have to try this one more time.

다시 한 번 해야 될 것 같습니다.

God! I am afraid I missed again.

이런. 또 놓쳤군요.

I will try one more time. I am sorry.

다시 한 번 해야 되겠습니다. 죄송합니다.

You have very tough veins. No good veins.

정맥이 좋지 않군요. 괜찮은 정맥이 없네요.

It'll hurt a bit. OK. I got it.

약간 아플 수 있습니다. 오케이. 됐습니다.

Now I am going to give you a shot in your buttock.

이제 엉덩이에 주사를 놓겠습니다.

Could you turn on your side?

옆으로 누워 줄래요?

It isn't proper posture.

자세가 적당하지 않네요.

Would you please lie down on the stomach?

엎드려 누우실래요?

Could you drop your pants and underwear?

바지와 속옷을 내려 주실래요?

I will sting a little bit. Take a relax.

약간 아플 수 있습니다. 진정하세요.

We are done.

다 됐습니다.

Press on this cotton.

이 솜을 누르세요.

If you feel any pain, just let me know.

통증이 있으면 제게 말해 주세요.

P : It really hurts.

정말 아프네요.

N : You can expect some soreness after shot.

주사를 맞고 나서 시릴 수 있습니다.

Using ice pack at the injection site for 20 minutes will reduce your pain.

20분 정도 주사 맞은 곳에 얼음찜질을 하면 통증이 줄어 들 것입니다.

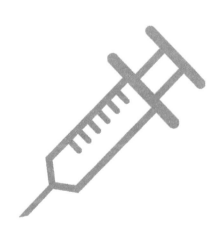

14. 약물 복용에 관한 설명들

Very Useful Expressions

1. It's time to take your pills.
   약 먹을 시간입니다.
2. Here is your medicine.
   여기 당신의 약이 있습니다.
3. I'll get you some medicines.
   약을 좀 드리겠습니다.
4. Take these medicines with plenty of water.
   이 약들을 많은 물과 함께 복용하세요.
5. Please take your medicine half an hour before your meal.
   식사 30분 전에 약을 복용하세요.
6. Take this medicine before meal.
   식전에 이 약을 드세요.
7. Take the medicine 30 minutes after meal.
   식후 30분 후에 드세요.
8. Take the medicine three times a day after meal.
   하루 세 번씩 식후에 약을 드세요
9. Take medicines every 12 hours.
   약들을 12시간마다 복용하세요.

10. Take medicines with every meal and at bedtime.

매 식사 때와 잠자기 전에 먹으세요.

11. Take pills about 30 minutes before you go to bed.

자기 30분 전에 약을 드세요.

12. Don't take on an empty stomach because it can irritate your stomach.

위를 자극하므로 빈속에는 먹지 마세요.

13. Did you take your medicine on time?

제 시간에 약을 드셨나요?

14. Medicine doesn't seem to be working.

약이 별로 효과가 없는 것 같습니다.

15. There may be side effects in the medicine.

약에 부작용이 있을 수 있습니다.

16. If you experience any side effects, stop taking it.

부작용이 있으면 먹지 마세요.

환자에게 약을 하루에 세 번 식후에 복용하도록 설명할 경우,

Take the medicine three times a day after meal. 라 하고,

두 번 복용은 twice a day,

식전 복용은 before meals,

공복 시 복용은 on an empty stomach,

많은 물과 함께 복용하라는 with plenty of water 를 사용한다.

약과 함께 물을 많이 마시라는 표현은

You need to drink a lot of water when you take the medicine.

You need to drink plenty of liquids with the medication.

약을 음식이나 뭔가를 먹은 후 드세요. 는

Take it after meals or with something in your stomach. 이다.

약을 제시간에 먹었느냐는

Did you take your medicine on time?

약이 효과를 나타낼 때까지 시간이 필요하다는

We have to give the medicine a little time to work.

약이 효과가 없다는 Medicine is not working.

그리고 약에 부작용이 있을 수 있다는

There may be side effects in the medicine. 이다.

환자에게 처방전을 줄 때는 Here is your prescription.

이 약이 당신의 증상을 완화 시켜줄 것입니다. 라는 표현은

Medication will help you get rid of the symptoms.

This medicines will relieve your symptom.

Your symptoms will wear off after taking the medicine.

처방전을 약국에 가져가세요. 는

Take the prescription to the pharmacy.

어느 약국에서든 약을 받을 수 있을 것입니다. 는

You can have filled at any pharmacy.

You can get it filled at any drug store. 라고 표현한다.

환자에게 약 용량을 바꾸지 마세요. 라고 말할 때는

Don't change the dosage of medication.

진통제를 복용할 경우, 술이나 담배를 금하세요. 는

Don't drink alcohol beverages or smoke

while taking pain medication. 로 표현한다.

Conversation

N : Good morning, Mr. Smith. I'll be looking after you this morning.

안녕하세요. 스미스씨. 오늘 오전은 제가 돌봐 드릴 것입니다.

P : Hello. You've got a great smile.

안녕하세요. 웃는 모습이 좋으시네요.

N : Thank you. How are you feeling today?

감사합니다. 오늘은 어떠세요?

P : Not so good actually.

좋지는 않네요.

I had a bad night sleep.

밤에 잠을 잘 못 잤네요.

And my operation site is really aching.

그리고 수술한 곳이 너무 아프네요.

N : I'm sorry to hear that.

저런, 그러세요?

Let me take a look.

제가 좀 볼게요.

I'd like to see if I can do anything about your pain.

통증을 제가 어떻게 할 수 있을지 볼게요.

Did you take your medicine on time?

제 시간에 약을 드셨나요?

P : Yes. Medicines seem to be not working.

네. 약들이 안 듣는 것 같아요.

N : It takes a little time to work.

효과가 있으려면 시간이 좀 걸립니다.

P : I can't stand it any more.

더 못 참겠습니다.

N : OK. I'll give you a shot of prn painkiller.

알겠습니다. 임시 진통제 주사를 놔 드릴게요.

There you go.

됐습니다.

I hope you are feeling more comfortable.

좀 더 좋아지길 바랍니다.

P : Thanks. I feel much better.

감사합니다. 좋아진 것 같아요.

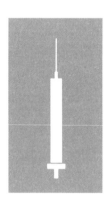

N : That's great.

잘 되었군요.

I need to go now.

이제 가봐야 합니다.

But if you need me, use the buzzer.

필요하면 벨을 누르세요.

See you soon.

좀 있다 볼게요.

94

15. 환자가 도움을 청했을 때

Very Useful Expressions

1. I am on my way. (I am coming. I'll be right there.)

   곧 갈게요.

2. I'll be there in a few minutes.

   몇 분 안에 가겠습니다.

3. What happened? (What's the matter?)

   무슨 일이죠?

4. How can I help you? Do you need anything?

   (What can I do for you?)

   (Is there anything else I can do for you?)

   무엇이 필요합니까?

5. Did you press the bell?

   벨을 누르셨나요?

6. Is anything bothering you?

   무슨 문제가 있나요?

7. Do you have pain?

   통증이 있나요?

8. In which part of your body do you feel the pain?

   몸 어느 부분이 아프세요?

9. When did the pain start?

언제 통증이 시작되죠?

10. Has the pain been getting worse?

통증이 더 악화되나요?

11. Does the pain come on at any particular time?

통증이 특정한 시간에 오나요?

12. I'll give you an injection to relieve the pain.

통증을 줄여주는 주사를 놔주겠습니다.

13. Does it still hurt now?

아직도 아프나요?

14. Didn't painkiller work?

진통제가 효과가 없던가요?

15. Doctor is with other patient right now.

의사선생님은 지금 다른 환자와 함께 있습니다.

16. I'll call the doctor.

의사선생님을 부를게요.

17. Doctor will come here and start your necessary treatment.

의사 선생님이 오셔서 필요한 치료를 해 줄 것입니다.

18. Doctor. Would you come immediately?

선생님 빨리 좀 와 주실래요?

19. Patient is having trouble breathing.

환자가 숨을 잘 쉬지 못합니다.

20. Patient is in a serious condition.

환자가 심각한 상태입니다.

21. The breathing difficulty has been going on for a couple
     of minutes.
    호흡곤란이 몇 분간 지속되었습니다.

22. Come quickly.
    빨리 와 주세요.

23. Residents are on call.
    레지던트 선생님들을 불렀습니다.

24. Doctor is gonna be here.
    의사선생님이 곧 이곳에 올 것입니다.

25. We will get a doctor to see you right away.
    지금 바로 선생님이 보시도록 하겠습니다.

26. Vitals are stable.
    활력징후는 괜찮습니다.

27. We need to move you into a treatment room.
    당신을 치료실로 옮겨야 합니다.

28. You'll need to have some test done.
    몇 가지 검사가 필요합니다.

29. It's necessary for you to get X-rays.
    방사선 검사가 필요합니다.

30. We would like to monitor you for the time being to
     make sure your are fine.
    당신이 괜찮은 지 모니터를 당분간 해야겠습니다.

31. Lie down for a while.
    당분간 누워 계세요.

32. We have to keep your room bright.

당신의 방을 밝게 하고 있어야 합니다.

33. Please keep the light on.

방의 불을 켜 두세요.

34. Is there anything I can do to make you feel comfortable?

당신을 편하게 해 줄 무언가가 필요하세요?

35. If you feel any discomfort, just let me know.

만약 불편한 느낌이 들면 저에게 알려 주세요.

저를 부르시려면 이 버튼을 눌러 주세요. 라는 표현은

If you want to call me, please press this button.

그리고 환자가 도움 벨을 눌렀을 경우 벨을 누르셨나요?

Did you push the bell?

Did you press the bell? Did you ring a bell? 로 물으면 되고,

무엇이 필요하세요? 무슨 일이죠?로 물어 볼 때는

What do you need? What do you want?

Do you need anything? What happened? What's the matter?

지금 즉시 처리하겠다는 말은

I'll take care of that right away.

조금 기다리세요, 제가 그 문제를 처리할게요.

Wait a minute. I'll take care of the problem.

의사를 부를게요. I'll call the doctor.

선생님이 이곳으로 오면 당신과 이야기할 수 있을 것입니다. 는

Doctor will come here and you can converse with doctor. 이다.

Conversation

N : Did you ring the bell?

벨을 누르셨나요?

What's the matter?

무슨 일이시죠?

Do you need anything?

무엇이 필요합니까?

P : I'd like to go to the bathroom.

화장실을 가고 싶어요.

N : Did you have a bowel movement in the morning?

아침에 화장실 가셨나요?

P : Yes.

네.

N : How many times did you have bowel movements today?

오늘 대변을 몇 번 보셨나요?

P : Twice. But I want to use the toilet again.

2번 갔어요. 그래도 또 화장실 가고 싶습니다.

N : OK. I'll help you.

알겠습니다. 도와드릴게요.

P : Thank you.

고마워요.

N : What color was your stool?

대변 색이 어떻던가요?

P : As usual, nothing special.

늘 그렇듯이, 별거 없어요.

N : Bed sheets are soaking wet.

침대 시트가 흠뻑 젖었군요.

I'll change that for you right away.

지금 바로 바꾸어 주겠습니다.

P : Thank you.

감사합니다.

N : Be careful not to catch a cold.

감기 걸리지 않게 조심하세요.

I'll give you extra blanket.

여분의 담요를 드리겠습니다.

P : I feel gloomy recently.

요즘 기분이 우울해요.

N : Old people tend to become emotional easily.

노인들은 쉽게 감정적으로 민감해 질 수 있습니다.

P : I don't have the strength to go around.

돌아다닐 힘이 없어요.

N : Try to use a wheelchair and get some sun.

휠체어를 타고 햇볕도 좀 쐬세요.

16. 병동에 걸려온 전화를 받을 때

Very Useful Expressions

1. A Hospital. Who is calling please?

   A 병원입니다. 누구시죠?

2. This is Nurse Kim.

   김 간호사입니다.

3. Hold on please.

   잠깐만 기다리세요.

4. Doctor. Phone is for you.

   선생님 전화 왔습니다.

5. Dr. Kim. There is a call from a Dr. Choi.

   김 선생님. 최 선생님에게서 전화 왔습니다.

6. Dr. Kim. Call on nurse station phone.

   김 선생님. 간호사 스테이션에 전화입니다.

7. He isn't available now.

   그는 전화를 받을 수 없습니다.

8. He is tied up with work.

   일에 얽매여 있습니다.

9. He is not here right now.

   그는 지금 여기에 없습니다.

10. Try to call again 30 minutes later.

    30분 뒤에 다시 전화해 보세요.

11. I'll tell him that you called.

    당신이 전화했다고 전해 드릴게요.

12. Probably he'll be gone for the rest of the day.

    아마도 오늘은 퇴근하신 것 같은데요.

13. May I take your message?

    메시지를 전해드릴까요?

14. If you leave a message, I'll pass it on to him.

    메시지를 남기면 전해줄게요.

15. Should I have him call you back?

    당신에게 전화를 드리라고 할까요?

16. I'll make sure he gets back to you.

    당신에게 전화를 드리라고 꼭 말할게요.

17. If you would like to speak with patient Mr. Kim,

    I'll transfer the line to him.

    김씨 환자분과 통화를 원하시면 전화를 돌려 드리겠습니다.

18. I'll connect you to the room 717.

    당신을 717호실로 연결해 드리겠습니다.

병원에 온 전화를 받을 때 소리가 잘 안 들릴 경우,

I have trouble hearing you.

상태가 좋지 않아 잘 안 들린다. 는

Connection isn't clear. Signal is bad. 로 표현하고,

환자나 보호자가 병원 전화를 사용하려고,

병원 전화를 잠깐 써도 되겠습니까?

Can I use hospital phone for a minute? 로 물어올 때,

부담 갖지 마세요. 는 Feel free. 로 대답하고,

공중전화가 어디에 있죠? Where is the pay phone? 라고 물으면,

저기 모퉁이에 있습니다.

Right over there. It's around the corner. 라 한다.

내선번호 -번 연결해 주세요. Please get me the extension -.

라는 외부 전화가 올 경우, 잠시만 기다리세요. 연결해 드릴게요.

One moment please. I'll connect you.

전화가 왔는데 바쁜 일을 처리하고 나중에 전화한다고 말할 때는

I am busy doing something.

I'll get back to you after doing rush-job. 라고 표현한다.

Conversation

P : Hello. May I speak to Dr. Kim?

　김 선생님 계신가요?

N : Who is calling please?

　누구시죠?

P : This is Mr. James.

　저는 제임스입니다.

　Is my doctor Kim available?

　담당의사 김 선생님과 통화할 수 있을까요?

N : Hold the line. Please.

잠깐만 기다리세요.

He can't come to the phone.

전화를 받을 수 없습니다.

He is participating in operation now.

지금 수술 중이십니다.

Would you like to leave a message?

메시지를 전해드릴까요?

If you leave a message, I'll pass it on to him.

메시지를 남기면 전해줄게요.

P : When will he be available?

언제쯤 통화가 가능할까요?

Will he come back soon?

곧 오시나요?

N : He'll be here on this afternoon maybe about 5 PM.

아마도 오후 5시경에는 있을 것 같습니다.

P : Could you tell him Mr. James called?

미스터 제임스가 전화했다고 전해주실래요?

N : Should I have him call you back?

당신에게 전화를 드리라고 할까요?

P : Thank you. Please tell him to call me back.

고맙습니다. 전화를 주시라고 전해주세요.

N : OK. I'll tell him that you called.

알겠습니다. 당신이 전화했다고 전해 드릴게요.

17. 수술 전 환자 체크에서 필요한 표현들

Very Useful Expressions

1. Did you notify family of your operation schedule?

   당신 가족들에게 수술 스케줄에 대해 설명했습니까?

2. The operation must be notified to the family.

   수술은 가족들에게 반드시 알려져야 합니다.

3. Call me when the family arrives.

   가족들이 오면 알려주세요.

4. I'd like to check your identity bracelet.

   신원 팔찌를 좀 확인해 보겠습니다.

5. Don't eat or drink anything after midnight prior to
   the day of surgery.

   수술 전날 자정 이후로는 아무 것도 먹거나 마시지 마세요.

6. I'd like to make sure that you had not had anything to eat.

   아무 것도 먹지 않았는지 확인하고 싶군요.

7. Fasting means that you cannot eat or drink anything for
   6 to 8 hours before surgery.

   금식이란 수술 전 6-8시간 동안 아무 것도 먹거나 마시지 않음을
   뜻합니다.

8. If you are taking any medicines, you should take your
   usual dose with a small sip of water before 6 am on the

day of surgery.

만약 어떤 약을 먹고 있으면 수술 당일 아침 6시에 약간의
물로 약을 먹어야 합니다.

9. You are allowed to drink a little water in the up to
   two hours before surgery.

   수술 전 2시간 전까지는 약간의 물을 마셔도 됩니다.

10. Do you have any loose teeth that could fall out?

    빠질지도 모르는 흔들리는 치아가 있나요?

11. Do you happen to wear contact lenses?

    혹시 콘택트 렌즈를 끼고 있나요?

12. You're going to move to operation room.

    수술실로 갈 것입니다.

13. Have you got any family here?

    여기에 가족 어느 분이 계시나요?

14. We'll insert urine catheter into your bladder.

    소변 도뇨관을 방광에 삽입하겠습니다.

15. It can make you feel uncomfortable, but it doesn't hurt.

    당신을 불편하게 하지만 아프지 않습니다.

16. Would you excuse us for a moment?

    잠시 자리를 좀 비켜 주실래요?

17. Everything is going to be fine.

    모든 것이 잘 될 것입니다.

18. Orderly. Take this patient to OR.

    오더리. 이 환자를 수술실로 데려가세요.

19. Be careful of his(her) arms (legs).

   팔(다리)을 조심하세요.

20. Watch the IV line.

   수액주사 줄을 조심하세요.

21. Let's move on my count. One. Two. Three.

   제가 셋 쉴 때 옮기세요. 하나, 둘, 셋.

22. Coming through. Clear the way.

   길 좀 비켜주세요.

23. Orderly took the patient to the operation room

   5 minutes ago.

   오더리가 환자를 5분 전에 수술실로 데려갔습니다.

24. Orderly. Please bring a bed to ward.

   오더리. 침대를 병실로 가져오세요.

문제를 치료하기 위해서는 수술이 필요합니다. 란 표현은

Surgery is necessary for you to treat this problem.

간단한 수술입니다. 는

It's a simple surgery.

크게 걱정할 필요 없습니다.

Don't worry. It's no big deal.

치료를 위해서는 수술이 최선의 선택입니다.

Surgery is the best choice for treatment.

많은 사람들이 이 수술을 받았습니다.

A lot of patients have had this surgery.

대부분의 환자들이 수술 후 좋아집니다.

Most patients get better after operation.

수술 전 금식이 필요합니다.

You need to fast before surgery.

수술 전날 자정 이후로는 아무 것도 먹거나 마시지 마세요.

Don't eat or drink anything after midnight

prior to the day of surgery.

신원 팔찌를 좀 확인해 보겠습니다. 는

May I check your ID bracelet?

I'd like to check your name(identity) bracelet. 로 표현한다.

Conversation

N : How long have you been fasting?

얼마나 금식을 하셨나요?

P : I didn't eat anything since last night.

어젯밤부터 아무 것도 먹지 않았습니다.

But I drank a glass of water at dawn.

헌데 새벽에 물 한잔 먹었습니다.

N : You are allowed to drink a little water up to two hours

before surgery.

수술 전 2시간 전까지는 약간의 물을 마셔도 됩니다.

OK. Do you have any loose teeth that could fall out?

알겠습니다. 빠질지도 모르는 흔들리는 치아가 있나요?

P : No.

없습니다.

N : Do you happen to wear contact lenses?

혹시 콘택트 렌즈를 끼고 있나요?

P : No. I have good sight.

아뇨. 시력이 좋은데요.

N : Are you nervous?

긴장이 되시나요?

P : Absolutely.

당연하죠.

Who doesn't feel afraid before surgery?

수술 전 어느 누가 두렵지 않겠습니까?

N : Calm yourself and take a deep breath.

진정하시고 숨을 크게 쉬어보세요.

P : OK.

알겠습니다.

N : A couple of hours may be necessary to give you fluids and

antibiotics and to prepare the operation.

수술전 수액과 항생제를 주고 또 수술 준비를 하기위해 1-2시간이

필요할 수 있습니다.

P : Will it hurt?

아플까요?

N : You will be under general anesthesia.

전신 마취를 할 것입니다.

You won't feel anything at all.

아무 느낌도 없을 것입니다.

P : How long does it take to finish?

끝나려면 얼마나 걸리죠?

N : Surgery will be over soon.

수술은 금방 끝납니다.

Don't worry. You feel better in a few days after an operation.

걱정 마세요. 수술 후 며칠 안에 좋아질 것입니다.

P : When does the operation start?

언제 수술이 시작되죠?

N : Calm down. You'll get an operation shortly.

진정하세요. 곧 수술을 받으실 겁니다.

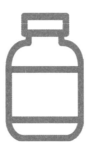

18. 수술을 마친 환자와의 대화

Very Useful Expressions

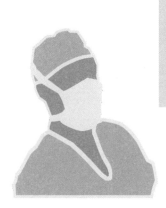

1. Stay calm. Relax.

   진정하세요.

2. You just have a major surgery.

   방금 당신은 큰 수술을 받으셨습니다.

3. Lie still.

   가만히 누워 계세요.

4. Take a deep breath, in and out.

   숨을 크게 들이마시고 내쉬세요.

5. The anesthetic hasn't worn off yet.

   아직 마취가 덜 깨서 그럽니다.

6. As time goes by, the effect will soon wear off.

   시간이 지남에 따라 곧 증상이 없어질 것입니다.

7. If you feel like vomiting, use this emesis basin.

   토할 것 같으면 이 농반을 사용하세요.

8. Don't put off oxygen mask. Put on.

   산소마스크를 벗지 마세요. 마스크를 쓰세요.

9. Pain medicines can relieve pain but it makes you drowsy.

   진통제가 통증을 줄여 주지만, 멍하게 만들 수가 있습니다.

10. You'll feel better in a couple of hours.
몇 시간 안에 좋아질 것입니다.
11. I'll be right over here if you need me.
필요하면 여기에 있을게요.
12. Did you break wind (fart)?
방귀를 뀌셨나요?
13. The first meal is a clear liquid diet.
처음 식사는 깨끗한 죽입니다.
14. If you need anything, just press the button.
필요한 것이 있으면 이 버튼을 눌러 주세요.
15. Take this medication after meal.
식사 후 이 약을 드세요.
16. It may be difficult to wash your face and brush teeth.
세수나 양치질이 어려울 것입니다.
17. You don't have to rush. Take your time.
서두르지 마세요. 천천히 하세요.
18. You can get help from caretaker.
간병인에게 도움을 받으세요.
19. If you are unable to walk, you have to use wheelchair.
걷지 못하시면 휠체어를 사용하셔야 합니다.
20. I will show you how to use a wheelchair.
휠체어를 어떻게 타는 지 가르쳐 드리겠습니다.
21. You can move around as much as you like.
당신이 하고 싶은 만큼 돌아다녀도 됩니다.

수술 후 마취를 깨우기 위해 필요한 표현들은,

입을 벌리고 크게 들이 쉬었다가 내 쉬세요.

Inhale fully with the mouth open and breathe out.

가능한 많은 공기를 들이 마시고 내 쉬세요.

You need to inhale and exhale as much air as possible.

깊게 숨을 쉬는 것은 수술 후 폐렴 예방에 도움이 됩니다.

Deep breathing helps prevent postoperative pneumonia.

침대에 앉아 있는 동안 약간 앞으로 숙여주세요.

Lean forward slightly while sitting in bed.

기침은 호흡기 객담을 배출하는데 도움을 줍니다.

Coughing is helpful to expel respiratory secretions.

입을 벌리고 깊게 숨을 들이 마신 다음,

한두 번 강하게 기침을 하세요.

With mouth open, take in a deep breath

and give one or two strong coughs. 등으로 표현한다.

수술 후 환자에게 방귀를 뀌었는지 물어 볼 때는

Did you fart?

Did you break wind?

Did you cut the cheese? 등으로 표현 할 수 있다.

Conversation

N : Take a deep breath, in and out.

숨을 크게 들이마시고 내쉬세요.

And cough in order to free your lungs of any possible fluid
due to the general anesthesia.

전신마취 때문에 당신의 폐에 생겼을지 모를 액체가 나오도록
기침을 하세요.

P : Cough! I feel dizzy.

콜록! 어지럽네요.

N : The anesthetic hasn't worn off yet. As time goes by,
the effect will soon wear off.

아직 마취가 덜 깨서 그럽니다.
시간이 지남에 따라 곧 증상이 없어질 것입니다.

P : I feel like vomiting.

토할 것 같아요.

N : Use this emesis basin.

이 농반을 사용하세요.

P : It gets very stuffy.

점점 더 답답하군요.

N : Don't put off oxygen mask. Put on.

산소마스크를 벗지 마세요. 마스크를 쓰세요.

P : I am feeling drowsy.

멍해지는 것 같아요.

N : Take a deep breath again.

숨을 다시 깊게 쉬세요.

With mouth open, take in a deep breath and give strong coughs.

입을 벌리고 깊게 숨을 들이 마신 다음, 강하게 기침을 하세요.

It will get better with time.

시간이 지남에 따라 좋아질 것입니다.

P : Did my surgery go well?

제 수술이 잘되었나요?

N : The surgery was fine. Operation was a success.

수술이 잘 되었습니다. 성공했습니다.

P : When can I eat?

언제 먹을 수 있죠?

N : You are allowed to eat when the stomach and intestines begin to function again.

위와 장의 기능이 돌아오면 먹을 수 있습니다.

P : Would I be able to eat solid food?

고형식을 먹을 수 있나요?

N : The first meal is a clear liquid diet.

처음 식사는 깨끗한 죽입니다.

If you tolerate liquid meal, the next meal usually is a regular diet.

죽을 먹고 괜찮으면 정상적인 음식이 나올 것입니다.

19. 운동이 필요한 환자와의 대화

Very Useful Expressions

1. Movement is good for you.

   움직이는 것이 당신에게 좋습니다.

2. Early ambulation helps you improve blood circulation, stimulate respiratory functions, and decrease the stasis of gas in the intestines.

   조기 보행은 혈액순환을 돕고, 호흡기능을 증가시키고, 장내 가스 정체를 감소시킵니다.

3. Early exercise is a good way to recover quickly after operation.

   조기 운동은 수술 후 빨리 회복하기 위한 좋은 방법입니다.

4. Are you having difficulty standing up?

   일어나시기 힘이 드세요?

5. Resume your normal physical activities as soon as possible.

   가능한 빨리 걷고 정상적인 활동을 시작하세요.

6. You can move around as much as you like.

   당신이 하고 싶은 만큼 돌아다녀도 됩니다.

7. Light exercise will improve your appetite and be helpful for deep sleep.

   가벼운 운동은 식욕을 일으키고 깊은 잠을 자게 해줍니다.

운동이 병에서 빨리 회복 시켜준다 라는 표현은

Exercise is a good way to recover quickly from illness.

매일 운동을 해야 된다는

You need to get some exercise every day.

30분 동안 걸어야 효과가 있다. 란

You need to walk for 30 minutes to have benefits.

운동이 당신의 몸을 튼튼하게 해 줄 것입니다. 란

Exercise will build up healthy body.

운동이 근육을 이완시키고, 잠을 잘 자게하고,

엔돌핀을 분비해 스트레스를 줄여준다는

Exercise can help you handle stress by relaxing tense

muscles, helping you sleep better and releasing endorphin.

콜레스테롤이나 지방이 많은 음식은 피하여야 한다는 표현은

You have to avoid any food containing

too much cholesterol or fat.

기름진 음식이나 설탕을 피하라는 표현은

You need to avoid highly greasy foods and sugar.

몸에 좋은 음식은 먹고 좋진 않은 음식은 피하라는 표현은

You need to eat healthy foods and avoid unhealthy foods.

신선한 과일이나 채소, 가공되지 않은 곡물, 단백질 등

올바른 식생활을 해야 된다는 표현은

You make sure that you eat the right foods like fresh fruits,

vegetables, whole grains and protein. 로 쓸 수 있다.

Conversation

N : Your symptoms have improved.

증상이 좋아졌습니다.

P : Can I walk?

걸을 수 있나요?

N : Yes. You can walk

네. 걸을 수 있습니다.

Actually movement is good for you.

사실 움직이는 것이 당신에게 좋습니다.

Resume your activities as soon as possible.

가능한 빨리 활동을 시작하세요.

Move around. Go here and there.

돌아다니세요. 이곳저곳을 다니세요.

P : When can I be discharged from the hospital?

언제 병원에서 퇴원할 수 있을까요?

N : You will be discharged from the hospital within 7 days after

the operation.

수술 후 7일 이내에 퇴원할 수 있을 것입니다.

And you are able to be back to your normal activities

within 2 weeks.

그리고 2주 이내에 정상 생활로 돌아 갈 수 있을 것입니다.

P : When can I play sports again?

언제 다시 스포츠를 할 수 있죠?

N : You are able to return to enjoy sports within four weeks

after the operation.

당신은 수술 후 4주 이내에 정상적인 스포츠를 즐길 수 있을 것입니다.

Do you exercise regularly?

규칙적으로 운동을 하시나요?

P : Sometimes. Walking, jogging, bicycling.

가끔씩요. 걷기, 조깅, 자전거 타기요.

But how can exercise help my diabetes?

그런데 운동이 어떻게 당뇨병에 도움을 주지요?

N : Exercise can help control your weight and lower your

blood sugar level.

운동은 당신의 몸무게를 조절해 주고 혈당도 줄여줍니다.

It also lowers your risk of disease and helps you feel better.

그리고 질병위험을 줄여주고 기분을 좀 더 좋게 만들어 줄 것입니다.

And actually exercise changes positively the way of your

body reacts to insulin.

그리고 사실 운동은 당신의 몸이 인슐린에 반응하는 것을 좋게

변화시켜 줍니다.

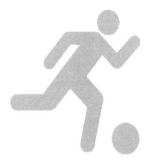

20. 낙상 방지를 위한 설명

Very Useful Expressions

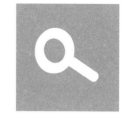

1. Was there a history of recent falls?
   최근에 낙상하신 적이 있나요?

2. We try to screen patients for falls risk and manage many
   of the risk factors.
   우리는 낙상 위험을 체크해 보고, 위험인자들을 처리하려고
   노력합니다.

3. Patients who have a high risk of falling will be checked
   regularly.
   낙상 위험이 높은 환자들은 규칙적으로 체크될 것입니다.

4. Family or Caretakers have to always stay with the patient
   if he(she) is at a high risk of falling.
   낙상 위험이 있을 경우 가족이나 간병인들은 항상 환자와 함께
   있어야 합니다.

5. Ask the nursing staff for help to go to the bathroom.
   화장실에 가고 싶다고 간호사들에게 알려주세요.

6. Ask for help when you need to get up.
   일어나고 싶으면 도움을 청하세요.

7. The bed should be in the lowest position and brakes on.
   침대는 낮추고 브레이크는 고정이 되어 있어야 합니다.

8. Take your time getting out of the bed.

　침대에서 나갈 때 시간을 충분히 갖으세요.

9. Sit at the edge of the bed for a few seconds before you get up.

　일어나기 전 침대 가장자리에서 몇 초간 앉아 있다가 일어나세요.

10. Wear nonslip slippers when you are up.

　서 있을 때는 미끄러지지 않는 슬리퍼를 신으세요.

11. You need to use a cane or walker.

　지팡이나 보행기를 사용하세요.

12. Use a shower chair.

　샤워 의자를 사용하세요.

13. Be careful, the bathroom floor is slippery.

　화장실 바닥이 미끄러우니 조심하세요.

14. Watch out. Watch your step.

　조심하세요. 발밑을 조심하세요.

15. Caretaker should stay with patients while the patient is in the bathroom.

　간병인은 환자가 화장실에 있는 동안도 같이 있어야 합니다.

16. Tell us if you have any concerns about your safety.

　안전상 불안한 점이 있으면 알려주세요.

17. Use the call button when you need help.

　도움이 필요하면 벨을 눌러 주세요.

인구의 고령화가 진행됨에 따라 병원에 입원해 있는
노인 환자들의 낙상 예방 교육이나 간호사들의
Safety Rounding (안전을 위한 회진)이 아주 중요하다.
보호자들에게 병원에 입원한 모든 노인들은 낙상 위험에 대해
확인되어야 합니다. 라고 설명할 때는
All older people who are admitted to hospital
should be screened for their falls risk.
인지부족 환자들은 쉽게 넘어집니다. 라는 표현은
Patients with cognitive impairment tend to fall easily.
병원 대부분의 낙상은 보지 못한 사이에 일어납니다.
Most falls in hospitals are unwitnessed.
그러므로 간병인이나 가족들이 항상 가까이서 지켜보아야 합니다.
Therefore carers, family members need for close monitoring.
간병인은 환자와 함께 앉아서 시간을 보내야 합니다.
Carers need to spend time sitting with the patient.
화장실 갈 때 도움을 청하세요.
Ask for help when you need to go to the bathroom.
보행기 사용이 필요합니다. You need to use a walker.
바닥에 물이 있으니 조심하세요. Floor is wet, be careful.
화장실 타일 바닥이 물에 젖어 미끄럽습니다.
Tiled floor in bathroom is wet with water, it's very slippery.
간병인은 항상 환자와 함께 있어야 합니다.
Caretaker has to always stay with the patient. 등으로 표현한다.

Conversation

P : My buttock is bruised and extremely sore.

엉덩이에 멍이 들고 아프네요.

N : How did you get hurt?

어떻게 다쳤나요?

P : I slipped on, and then fell down in the hallway.

오늘 아침 미끄러져 복도에서 넘어졌어요.

N : Oh, that's a pity.

저런, 안 되었군요.

Falls are very common in older people.

노인들에게 낙상은 매우 흔하게 발생합니다.

One of the most serious fall injuries is a broken hip.

가장 심각한 손상이 고관절 골절입니다.

It is hard to recover from a hip fracture

고관절 골절에서 회복하기가 어렵습니다.

P : As I get older, I am always afraid of falling.

나이가 드니 항상 넘어질 까 걱정이 됩니다.

N : Falls can result in bone fracture.

낙상은 골절이 될 수 있습니다.

Please, be careful.

제발 조심하세요.

P : Aging can cause me to become fearful and making it difficult to

stay active.

나이를 먹은 것이 나를 두렵게 하고 활동적이지 못하게 합니다.

N : Yes. As we age, most of us lose some strength and balance.

나이가 들면 우리들 대부분은 힘과 균형을 잃습니다.

It makes easier to fall.

쉽게 넘어지죠.

Bones become brittle.

뼈들도 잘 부러지고요.

P : I have difficulty walking and arising from a chair.

의자에서 일어나기 어렵습니다.

I am holding onto walls when walking.

걸을 때 벽을 잡고 다닙니다.

N : You need to use a cane or walker.

지팡이나 보행기를 사용하세요.

And take your time getting out of the bed.

그리고 침대에서 나갈 때 시간을 충분히 갖으세요.

Sit at the edge of the bed for a few seconds before you get up.

일어나기 선 침대 가장자리에서 몇 초간 앉아 있다가 일어나세요.

You need to wear nonslip slippers when you are up or walk.

서 있거나 걸을 때는 미끄러지지 않는 슬리퍼를 신을 필요가 있습니다.

Reducing the risks of falling is a great way to help old people

stay healthy and independent as long as possible.

낙상 위험을 낮추는 것이 노인들을 오랫동안 건강하고 독립적으로

살 수 있게 도와줍니다.

P : How do I become a more careful at home?

집에서는 어떻게 더 조심해야 하죠?

N : Increase lighting throughout the house.

집안의 불빛을 밝게 해주세요.

Make sure there are secure rails.

안전 손잡이가 있게 해야 합니다.

Install grab bars in the bathroom and near the toilet.

화장실이나 화장실 근처에 손잡이 바가 있어야 합니다.

Bathroom floors should be skidproof.

화장실 바닥은 미끄러짐 방지 타일이어야 합니다.

And get rid of things you could trip over.

그리고 걸려 넘어질 수 있는 것들을 치우세요.

Make sure to follow our advice.

저희 말들을 꼭 따라주세요.

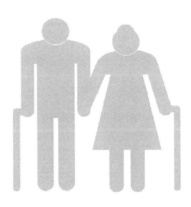

21. 환자 간병인에게 손 씻는 방법 가르쳐 주기

Very Useful Expressions

1. You need to wash your hands frequently.

   손을 자주 씻으셔야 합니다.

2. Your hands should be cleaned immediately after direct contact patient.

   환자와 접촉하고 나면 바로 즉시 손을 씻으셔야 합니다.

3. Rub your palms together with your fingers closed, and then together with fingers interlaced.

   손가락을 붙이고 손바닥을 문지른 다음 손가락 사이를 함께 비비세요.

4. Interlock your fingers and rub the hand.

   손가락을 깍지 낀 다음 문지르세요.

5. Clasp your thumb in your other palm and rub in a rotational motion, then switch hands, vice versa.

   한쪽 엄지손가락을 반대쪽 손바닥으로 잡고 돌리면서 문지른 다음, 손을 바꾸고 그 반대로 하세요.

6. Rinse your hands well under running water and dry your hands using a clean towel.

   흐르는 물에 손을 잘 씻고 깨끗한 수건으로 닦으세요.

자주 손을 씻는 것이 질병 확산을 방지하는 가장 좋은 방법입니다.

라는 표현은

Frequent hand－washing is one of the best ways

to avoid spreading illness.이고,

이 세정제를 사용하세요.

Use this hand sanitizer. Use this hand cleanser.

사람이나 물건을 만질 때 손에 세균들이 모아집니다.

As you touch people and objects,

you accumulate germs on your hands.

눈이나 코, 입을 통해 이 세균들이 전염됩니다.

You can infect yourself with these germs

by touching your eyes, nose or mouth.

손을 자주 씻는 것이 세균 전파를 막아줍니다.

Washing your hands frequently can help prevent from

transferring of germs. 등으로 표현한다.

Conversation

N : Are you tired of caring the patient?

환자를 돌보느라 피곤하지 않으세요?

P : It's obligatory for family to care their patient.

가족들이 환자를 돌보는 것은 당연한 것이죠.

N : Do you wash your hands frequently?

손을 자주 씻으시나요?

127

Your hands should be cleaned immediately after direct contact patient.

환자와 접촉하고 나면 바로 즉시 손을 씻으셔야 합니다.

P : I try to, but it's easier said than done.

노력은 하는데 말하기보다 행하는 것이 쉽지는 않더군요.

By the way, can you explain to me about a proper hand washing?

그나저나 어떻게 적절하게 손을 씻어야 하는지 설명해 주실래요?

N : No problem. Wet hands with water, apply soap and wash your hands for about 15 seconds.

알겠습니다. 손을 적시고 비누를 묻힌 다음 15초 동안 손을 씻으세요.

P : Can you explain in more detail?

좀 더 자세하게 설명해 주실래요?

N : OK. First, begin rubbing your palms together with your fingers closed, then together with fingers interlaced.

그러죠. 먼저 손가락을 붙이고 손바닥을 문지른 다음 손가락 사이를 함께 비비세요.

Next, move your right palm over left dorsum with interlaced fingers and rub in between your fingers. Vice versa.

그리고 다음은 우측 손바닥을 반대 손등으로 가져가 손가락 사이까지 문지르고 그 반대로 똑같이 하세요.

P : Like this?

이렇게요?

N : Yes. And interlock your fingers and rub the back of them by turning your wrist in a half circle motion.

네. 그리고 손가락을 모으고 손목을 약간 회전시키며 손가락 등을
문지르세요.

Clasp your left thumb in your right palm and rub in a rotational
motion, then switch hands, vice versa.

좌측 엄지손가락을 우측 손바닥으로 잡고 돌리면 문지른 다음,
손을 바꾸고 그 반대로 하세요.

P : It's not as easy as I thought.

생각한 만큼 쉽지는 않군요.

N : If it becomes a habitual, it'll be a piece of cake.

일단 습관화 되면 식은 죽 먹기입니다.

And finally scrub the inside of your right hand backwards and
forwards with your left clasped fingers and vise versa.

Rinse your hands well under running water and dry your hands
using a clean towel.

그리고 마지막으로 좌측 구부린 손가락들로 우측의 손바닥을 앞뒤로
문지르고, 반대 손도 똑같이 한 다음, 흐르는 물에 손을 잘 씻고
깨끗한 수건으로 닦으세요.

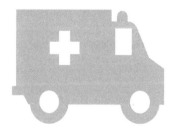

22. 병동에서 필요한 여러 가지 표현들

Very Useful Expressions

1. Right now all the beds are full.
   지금은 모든 침대가 다 찼습니다.

2. We'll get you a bed as soon as one is available.
   빈 침대가 생기면 바로 알려드리겠습니다.

3. We have one open bed.
   침대 한 개가 비어 있습니다.

4. We are going to exchange bed sheets to a new one.
   침대시트를 새것으로 바꾸어주겠습니다.

5. Your bed sheet is wet.
   당신의 시트가 젖었군요.

6. We will change your bed sheet right now.
   바로 지금 시트를 교환해드리겠습니다.

7. Excuse me for a second. I'll be right back.
   잠깐 실례할게요. 곧 돌아오겠습니다.

8. Sorry to keep you waiting.
   기다리게 해서 죄송합니다.

9. Would you please step aside for a moment?
   잠시만 옆으로 비켜주실래요?

130

10. Did you have a bowel movement and urination?

대변과 소변을 보셨나요?

11. We need to put a catheter in to get urine.

소변을 받으려 도뇨관을 넣을 것입니다.

12. You might be a bit uncomfortable.

약간 불편 하실 겁니다.

13. It won't take long.

오래 걸리지 않을 것입니다.

14. It won't hurt much.

많이 아프지는 않습니다.

15. I'll measure your urine output.

소변 양을 측정하겠습니다.

16. I'm here to change your bedpan.

소변기를 바꾸어주려고 왔습니다.

17. We will change your diaper.

기저귀를 갈아드리겠습니다.

18. I'll help you put on your clothes.

옷 입는 것을 도와 드릴게요.

19. Can I give Mr. Kim more prn injection?

김씨에게 prn 주사를 더 주어도 될까요?

20. May I check your identity bracelet?

신원확인 팔찌를 좀 확인해 보겠습니다.

21. Your IV line is not properly connected.

혈관주사가 잘못 연결되었군요.

22. We have to sterilize your wound.

상처를 소독해야 합니다.

23. Let me take a look.

잠깐 볼게요.

24. Please lie still. Don't move.

가만히 누워 계세요. 움직이지 마세요.

25. Would you like to sit up?

앉아 주실래요?

26. It seems to be all right.

괜찮은 것 같군요.

27. The food isn't warm enough?

음식이 충분히 따뜻하지 않나요?

28. The food isn't cooked properly?

음식이 잘못 요리되었나요?

29. We will give a report to the nutritionist for improving

the taste.

맛을 개선하라고 영양사에게 말하겠습니다.

30. You'll need to have some test done.

몇 가지 검사가 필요합니다.

31. You need to get an X-ray.

X-ray를 찍어야 합니다.

32. You'll be going to get X-rays shortly.

곧 X-ray를 찍을 것입니다.

33. If you need anything, push the button
    and I'll come right away.

필요하면 버튼을 누르세요. 바로 오겠습니다.

34. Would you please keep the noise down?

소음을 좀 줄여주실래요?

35. Please be mindful not bothering other patients.

다른 환자분들이 신경 쓰이지 않게 조심해 주세요.

36. Electric outlet is not working?

전기 콘센트가 작동이 안 되나요?

37. Is TV not working?

TV 작동이 안 되나요?

38. The TV is broken?

TV가 고장이 났나요?

39. The toilet is blocked?

화장실이 막혔나요?

40. Hot water is not coming out?

뜨거운 물이 안 나오나요?

41. Toilet paper is gone?

화장지가 없나요?

42. We will give a report on it to the management department.

그것에 대해 관리과에 보고를 할 것입니다.

43. It will take time to fix it.

고치려면 시간이 걸립니다.

45. Don't do things like that. It's very annoying.

그런 짓을 하지 마세요. 신경이 거슬리네요.

46. We need to get written permission, if you want to go out.

외출 하려면 서면허가증이 필요합니다.

47. My shift is over.

제 근무시간이 끝났습니다.

48. I need to leave(go) now. (I guess I should go.)

(I really must get going. It's time for me to go)

지금 가야 할 것 같습니다.

49. I'll be back tomorrow.

내일 다시 오겠습니다.

50. See you next time.

다음에 뵙겠습니다.

병동 업무 중 환자나 보호자들과 마찰이 있을 경우,

자신의 감정과 입장을 조심스레,

논리적으로 표현할 필요가 있는데, 예로써

우리는 감정적으로 힘든 일을 하고 있습니다.

We work in an emotionally intense kind of field.

환자를 돌보는 방법과, 개인 간의 관계가 중요하다고 생각합니다.

We think interpersonal relation is an important part of

how we take care of our patients.

간호사들은 환자치료 팀에서 아주 중요한 일원입니다.

Nurses are important members of a patient's treatment team.

환자들을 돌보는 데 많은 역할을 하고 있습니다.

We have many roles in the care of patients.

간호사들은 환자 치료의 최전방에 있습니다.

Nurses are in the front of patient care.

그러나 우리를 좌절 시키는 일들이 많습니다.

But there are many times when we get so angry or frustrated.

당신이 우리를 흥분하게 하고 좌절하게 만듭니다.

You have really irritated us and frustrated us.

왜 이렇게 행동하시나요?

Why would you behave like this?

저를 괴롭히지 마세요. Stop bothering me.

저는 항상 환자가 이유가 있고, 정당하다고 생각합니다.

I always think patients are reasonable and decent.

그런데 당신의 행동은 그것을 다시 생각하게 하는군요.

But your behaviors give me chance to rethink about it.

진정하세요. You need to calm down.

그래서 합리적으로 대화를 나누고 싶습니다.

So I'd like to have a conversation reasonably.

같은 말들을 사용할 수 있다.

병동에서 환자가 자꾸 많은 말들로 일을 하는데 불편할 경우,

말을 끊어서 미안해요.

I'm sorry to cut you off.

지금 매우 바쁩니다.

I'm very busy at the moment.

다른 환자를 보아야 합니다. 미안합니다.

I've got another patient. Excuse me.

라고 말하며 피하는 것도 하나의 방법이다.

Conversation

N : How was your visit with family?

가족 방문은 좋았습니까?

P : Very good.

아주 좋았습니다.

N : That's great.

잘 되었군요.

We want you to get well as soon as possible.

우리는 당신이 되도록 빨리 회복되시기를 원합니다.

We will do everything we can to help.

도울 수 있는 것은 다 할 것입니다.

P : Thank you.

감사합니다.

Staying in hospital is very difficult for me.

병원에 있는 것이 너무 힘들군요.

N : Are you bored?

지루하시죠?

P : Yes. It's so boring.

정말 지루하군요.

N : Be patient. You will be discharged soon.

조금만 참으세요. 곧 퇴원을 하실 겁니다.

P : I am dying to see my puppy.

강아지가 보고 싶어 죽겠네요.

N : Have you any pets at home?

집에 애완동물을 기르고 있나요?

P : Yes. A little Maltese.

네 작은 말티즈입니다.

N : Who is taking care of the puppy?

누가 강아지를 돌보고 있죠?

P : My neighbors.

이웃사람들이 돌보고 있습니다.

N : Flu season is upon us.

독감 계절이 왔네요.

Be careful not to catch a cold after discharge.

퇴원 후 감기에 안 걸리게 조심하세요.

P : How can I boost my immunity?

어떻게 제 면역을 높일 수가 있죠?

N : Regular exercise, sufficient sleep and healthy foods are going to keep you from getting sick.

규칙적인 운동과 충분한 잠, 건강식이 잘 아프지 않게 해줄 것입니다.

P : Healthy food?

건강식 말인가요?

N : Yes. What you eat does matter.

예. 먹는 것이 관련됩니다.

P : What food is good for common cold?

감기에 좋은 음식이 뭐죠?

N : The ideal way to get healthy foods is to eat sufficient protein and variable fruits and vegetables.

건강식이란 충분한 단백질과 다양한 과일, 채소들을 먹는 것입니다.

P : Can Vitamin C prevent me from catching the flu?

비타민 C가 독감 걸리는 것을 예방해 주나요?

N : Taking vitamins is not going to supercharge your immune system.

비타민을 먹었다고 면연력이 아주 높아지지는 않습니다.

Vitamin C doesn't seem to reduce the incidence of colds, though it might be helpful for tired people.

비타민C가 비록 피곤한 사람들에게 도움을 줄지는 몰라도 감기 걸리는 빈도를 줄여주지는 않습니다.

Eat more fruits and vegetables.

과일과 채소를 많이 드세요.

They have abundant vitamins and anthocyanin.

그것들은 풍부한 비타민들과 안토시아닌을 가지고 있습니다.

Natural foods help you keep your health.

자연 음식이 당신의 건강을 지키는데 도움을 줍니다.

23. 병원에서 환자가 퇴원할 때

Very Useful Expressions

1. You will be discharged soon if symptoms are improved.

   증상이 호전되면 곧 퇴원을 하실 것입니다.

2. Operation went well, and soon you will be discharged
   from the hospital.

   수술이 잘되었습니다. 그래서 곧 병원에서 퇴원 하실 것입니다.

3. Are you supposed to go home today?

   오늘 퇴원을 하시나요?

4. Please, go through the discharge procedure at the front
   desk on the first floor.

   일층 계산대에 가서 퇴원 수속을 밟으십시오.

5. Have you finished check out process?

   퇴원 수속을 마치셨나요?

6. Do you need a medical certificate & confirmation of
   hospitalization care?

   진단서와 입원확인서가 필요하십니까?

7. Do you need a doctor's note and copies of test results?

   의사 소견서와 검사 결과 복사본이 필요하십니까?

8. Here are your medications for 14 days.

   여기 당신의 14일분의 약들이 있습니다.

9. Please take your medicine on time.

정해진 시간에 약을 복용하세요.

10. Your follow up appointment is −.

당신의 재진 날짜가 - 입니다.

11. Come to the outpatient clinic on a given day.

정해진 날짜에 외래로 오십시오.

12. You are yet weak,

so I am concerned with your health care after discharge.

아직 당신이 약해서 퇴원 후 건강이 걱정이 됩니다.

13. If rehabilitation treatment are required,

arrangements must be made.

만약 재활 치료가 필요하면 적절한 곳을 알아보셔야 합니다.

14. If care cannot be provided at home after your discharge,

it is important to arrange for skilled nursing care in

care facility.

퇴원 후 집에서 간병이 이루어지지 않으면 전문 간호사의 도움이

필요한 요양원을 알아보시는 것도 좋습니다.

15. Parking will be free for up to 8 hours.

주차장은 8시간까지 무료입니다.

병동에서 환자와 상담을 할 때 필요한 표현들을 간단히 살펴보면,

당신의 고민을 이해합니다.

I can understand your distress.

저에게 어떤 것이든 말하세요.

I want you to talk to me about anything.

당신의 마음을 안정시키세요.

You need to calm yourself.

당신의 가족에게 말하세요.

Try to talk with your family.

그들이 당신을 돕고 치료에 대한 걱정을 줄여줄 것입니다.

They will help you and relieve anxiety about the treatment.

도움이 될 만한 게 있으면 좋겠군요.

I wish there is something I could do to help.

당신이 좋아질 것이라고 생각합니다.

I think you'll be fine.

우리가 당신을 잘 돌봐드릴 것입니다.

We'll take very good care of you. 등을 적절히 사용할 수 있다.

Conversation

N : Your hospital stay has ended.

병원에 게시는 것이 이제 끝났습니다.

P : Really? I am very glad to hear that.

정말요? 그 말을 들으니 매우 기쁘군요.

When can I get out of the hospital?

언제 병원을 나갈 수 있죠?

N : You will be informed of your approximate discharge time.

퇴원 시간을 알려 줄 것입니다.

If you have concerns about the discharge procedure,

please discuss them with adminstration staff.

퇴원 수속에 대해 상의할 것이 있으면 원무과 직원과 상의 하십시오.

P : Thank you for everything you have done for me.

저에게 대해 주신 모든 것에 감사드립니다.

N : Don't mention it.

천만에요.

That's what I have to do.

제가 할 일인데요.

I will explain about your continuing health care needs.

당신에게 지속적인 건강관리에 대해 설명해 드리겠습니다.

You need to have medications to take and follow-up

appointments will be arranged.

먹어야 할 약들을 받을 것이고, 다음 진료 시간을 예약해 줄 것입니다.

And for your safety, make arrangements for your trip home.

그리고 당신의 안전을 위해 집에 가실 계획을 세우셔야 합니다.

P : Age is nothing but a number.

나이는 숫자에 불과합니다.

I can handle all by myself.

모든 것을 혼자 할 수 있습니다.

N : Your family or friend have to escort you to your home.

그리고 당신 가족이나 친구가 반드시 집까지 데려다 주어야 합니다.

P : OK. As you wish.

알겠습니다. 당신이 원하는 대로 하죠.

What should I be careful after discharge from the hospital?

병원에서 퇴원 후 무엇을 조심해야 하나요?

N : Your doctor will explain about it.

담당 선생님이 설명해 주실 것입니다.

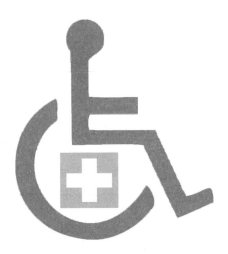

24. 입원환자의 간호 정보 조사지

PATIENT ADMISSION FORM
(BASIC MEDICAL QUESTIONS FOR INPATIENT)

NAME : FIRST   LAST
BIRTH DATE :
AGE :   SEX : MALE, FEMALE
ADDRESS :

1. REASON FOR ADMISSION OR DIAGNOSIS :

2. PRESENT ILLNESS

DO YOU HAVE DIABETES?
DO YOU HAVE HYPERTENSION?
DO YOU HAVE HEPATITIS (A, B, C)
    OR LIVER DISEASE?
DO YOU HAVE ANY GASTRIC PROBLEMS?
DO YOU HAVE ANY HEART PROBLEMS?
DO YOU HAVE ANY LUNG OR CHEST CONDITIONS?
DO YOU HAVE ANY BOWEL PROBLEMS?
DO YOU HAVE ANY KIDNEY

OR BLADDER PROBLEMS?

DO YOU HAVE ANY ALLERGY?

DO YOU SUFFER FROM ANY OTHER PROBLEM?

3. MEDICATION HISTORY

DO YOU TAKE ANY MEDICATIONS?

DO YOU TAKE ANTI−COAGULANT

     OR BLOOD THINNING MEDICATIONS?

DO YOU TAKE SLEEPING OR ANXIETY TABLETS?

4. HEALTH LIFE STYLE

DO YOU DRINK ALCOHOL?

HOW MUCH ALCOHOL DO YOU DRINK?

HOW MANY STANDARD DRINKS EACH DAY?

DO YOU SMOKE?

HOW MUCH DO YOU SMOKE?

HOW MANY CIGARETTES PER DAY?

HAVE YOU SMOKED IN THE PAST?

NUMBER OF YEARS :   , YEAR CEASED :

HOW OFTEN DO YOU EXERCISE?

DO YOU GET SHORT OF BREATH, CHEST PAIN

     OR PALPITATIONS AFTER EXERCISE?

HAVE YOU HAD A COLD OR FLU RECENTLY?

ARE YOU, OR COULD YOU BE, PREGNANT?

    (FOR WOMAN)

DO YOU HAVE ANY MOBILITY PROBLEMS?

    (arthritis, back pain, leg weakness)

DO YOU USE ANY MOBILITY AIDS?

    STICK / CRUTCHES / WHEELCHAIR (please circle)

DO YOU HAVE ANY HEARING PROBLEMS?

HEARING AIDS? LEFT,   RIGHT

DO YOU HAVE ANY PROBLEMS WITH YOUR VISION?

    (limited, cataracts, glaucoma)

DO YOU WEAR GLASSES?

    CONTACT LENSES ?

5. REVIEW FOR OPERATION

HAVE YOU EVER HAD AN OPERATION?

HAVE YOU EVER HAD AN ANAESTHETIC BEFORE?

HAVE YOU EVER HAD ANY PROBLEMS WITH
    ANAESTHETICS?

HAVE YOU EVER HAD A BLOOD TRANSFUSION?

DO YOU HAVE DIFFICULTY OPENING YOUR MOUTH
    WIDE OR HAVE LIMITED NECK MOVEMENT?

DO YOU HAVE ANY BROKEN, OR LOOSE TEETH?

PATIENT DECLARATION :

TO THE BEST OF MY KNOWLEDGE,
THE INFORMATION I HAVE PROVIDED IS TRUE
AND CORRECT.

PATIENT (OR PARENT/GUARDIAN) NAME :

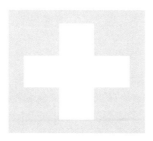

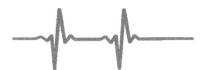

My Intuition guides me in what I do.

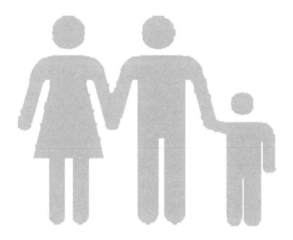

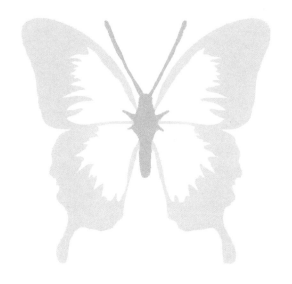

Part II
Hospital Departments Services

제 2부
병원 전문과목별 서비스
(외래 및 분과)

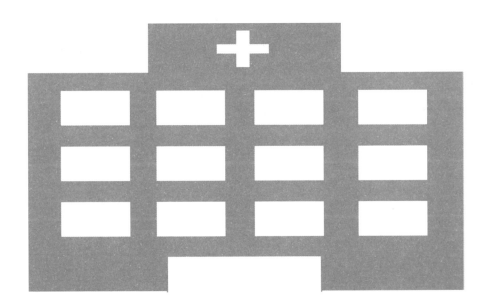

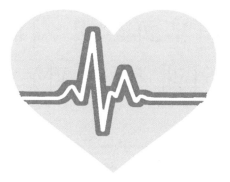

25. 진료실 외래에서 필요한 표현들

Very Useful Expressions

1. May I help you?
   무엇을 도와드릴까요?

2. Do you want to check in?
   접수를 원하시나요?

3. Please register at the reception desk in the main entrance lobby.
   정문 로비에 있는 접수처에 가서 접수해 주세요.

4. Please register at the front desk.
   앞에서 접수해 주세요.

5. Do you have a reservation?
   예약을 하셨나요?

6. Who is your doctor?
   담당 선생님이 누구시죠?

7. Do you have a consultation request?
   진료의뢰서를 가지고 있나요?

8. What seems to be the problem?
   무슨 문제가 있으시죠?

9. Is there a doctor you want to see?
   보시길 원하는 선생님이 계십니까?

제 2 부

10. Who would you like to see?

어느 선생님을 원하세요?

11. Do you want to see Dr. Lim?

임선생님을 원하세요?

12. What's your name?

이름이 어떻게 되지요?

13. How do you spell your name?

철자를 말해 줄래요?

14. What's your date of birth?

생일이 언제이지요?

15. I would like to verify your identity.

당신의 신원을 확인하고 싶군요.

16. Do you have any identification card?

어떤 신분증이 있나요?

17. Your appointment is 9 O'clock.

당신의 예약은 9시입니다.

18. Please wait in the waiting room.

대기실에서 기다려 주세요.

19. Take a seat over there and I'll let you know.

저기에 앉아 계시면 알려드리겠습니다.

20. Please have a seat until you are called.

부르실 때까지 앉아 계세요.

21. You need to go to the restroom before examination.

검사 전에 화장실을 다녀오세요.

22. Down this hallway.

　　이 복도를 따라 가세요.

23. Rest room is around the corner.

　　화장실은 모통이에 있습니다.

24. Since you arrived late, you have to wait to avoid delaying
other patients.

　　늦게 오셨기 때문에 다른 환자가 늦어지지 않도록 기다리셔야
합니다.

25. Sorry to have kept you waiting.

　　기다리게 해서 죄송합니다.

26. You will see a doctor a little later.

　　잠시 뒤 의사 선생님을 볼 것입니다.

27. It's your turn. Doctor will call you soon.

　　당신 차례입니다. 의사 선생님이 곧 부르실 겁니다.

28. Please come in and have a seat.

　　안으로 들어오셔서 자리에 앉으세요.

29. After paying at the reception desk, go to the X-ray
and blood lab.

　　접수처에서 계산을 한 다음에 X-ray실과 혈액 검사실로 가세요.

30. Follow the yellow line to the X-ray department.

　　방사선과로는 노란색을 따라 가세요.

31. Follow the arrows on the wall.

　　벽에 있는 화살표를 따라 가세요.

32. Follow the red line.
빨간색을 따라 가세요.

33. Come this way, please.
이쪽으로 오세요.

34. I'll show you to laboratory room.
임상병리실로 안내해 드리겠습니다.

35. You can leave when you are done.
다 끝나시면 가셔도 됩니다.

36. Please come here again and wait for a while.
이곳으로 다시 오셔서 잠시만 기다려 주십시오.

37. You will hear the result after a while.
잠시 뒤 결과를 들을 것입니다.

38. The prescription is for 14 days.
처방전은 14일분입니다.

39. You can fill this prescription at any pharmacy.
어느 약국에서나 약을 살 수 있습니다.

40. I'll make a follow-up appointment for you.
다음 진료 예약을 해드리겠습니다.

41. What date do you want?
어는 날짜를 원하시죠?

42. We have -, at 2 PM open.
-일 오후 2시가 비어있군요.

43. Will that be a good time?
괜찮습니까?

44. 3 PM is filled.

3시는 예약이 다 예약되었습니다.

45. 3:20 PM open.

3시 20분이 비어있습니다.

46. Will you take it?

이것으로 예약하시겠습니까?

47. Your appointment is -.

당신의 예약은 - 입니다.

48. See you then.

그날 뵙겠습니다.

49. The doctor told you need hospitalization.

의사선생님이 당신은 입원이 필요하다고 하십니다.

50. You need to be admitted to the hospital today.

오늘 병원에 입원하셔야 합니다.

51. Please go to the admission desk and check in.

입원계로 가서 수속해 주세요.

52. Please understand that the hospital has to find the appropriate bed for you.

병원에서 당신에게 맞는 병실 침대를 찾아야 하는 점을 이해해 주십시오.

53. This may take time.

이것은 시간이 걸릴지도 모릅니다.

54. It will take many hours.

몇 시간 걸립니다.

55. You have to wait until someone is discharged.

다른 분이 퇴원하기 전까지 기다리셔야 합니다.

56. Which type of room do you prefer?

몇 인실을 원하시나요?

57. If you want a private room, you may be expected to pay the additional fees.

1인실을 원하시면 추가 비용이 발생합니다.

58. You should give your valuables to your family.

귀중품은 가족들에게 맡기십시오.

59. Personal items like a gown, towel and slippers will be provided by the hospital.

병원 가운이나 수건, 슬리퍼는 병원에서 줄 것입니다.

60. You need to buy personal toiletries and daily necessaries at hospital convenience store.

세면도구나 생활용품들을 병원 매점에서 사셔야 합니다.

61. A nurse is assigned to you and responsible for your care.

담당 간호사가 배정되고 당신을 돌보아 줄 것입니다.

62. You will be under the care of the nurses after admission.

입원 후 간호사들이 돌보아 줄 것입니다.

Conversation

N : May I help you?

무슨 일로 오셨죠?

P : My child is running a fever.

아이가 열이 납니다.

N : How long has he had a fever?

열이 나는 지 얼마나 되었나요?

P : He has had a fever all night and will not eat.

밤새 열이 나고 먹질 않습니다.

We need help immediately.

빨리 좀 도와주세요.

N : I would like to take his weight, height, temperature and

blood pressure.

아이의 몸무게, 키, 체온과 혈압을 측정해야 되겠습니다.

Hi, sweetie, take off your shoes and stand on the scales.

아가야, 안녕, 신발을 벗고 체중계에 서 줄래?

Stand up here, weighing machine.

이곳에 서줄래? 체중계야.

We'll see how heavy you are.

얼마나 무거운 지 볼게.

I wonder how tall you are.

키가 얼마나 큰 지 궁금하구나.

Could you come and stand over here?

이곳으로 와서 서 줄래?

I'll check your height.

키를 측정할게.

Stand straight.

똑바로 서줄래?

I'll measure you now.

지금 잴거야.

You may step down.

내려와도 돼.

Put on your shoes.

신발을 신어도 돼.

Sit over there.

저기 앉을래?

I'll take your temperature.

체온을 잴게.

May I take your blood pressure?

혈압을 잴까?

We are all finished now.

이제 다 끝났어.

Have a seat in the waiting area for a moment.

대기실에서 잠시 만 기다려 주세요.

Doctor will be with you in a few minutes.

잠시 뒤 선생님을 뵙게 되실 겁니다.

Finished?

끝났나요?

P : He has got flu.

독감에 걸렸더군요.

Is there anything else that I need to take care of?

조심해야 될 것들이 있나요?

N : We want you to monitor his temperature.

그의 체온을 모니터 해 주세요.

P : How often should I check it?

얼마나 자주 체크해야 하죠?

N : Once every four hours.

4시간에 한 번 해주세요.

And doctor want to have a look at your kid again after 2 days.

그리고 선생님이 아이를 이틀 뒤에 다시 진료하길 원하십니다.

Make sure you visit the hospital the day after tomorrow.

모레 병원에 꼭 오세요.

제 2 부

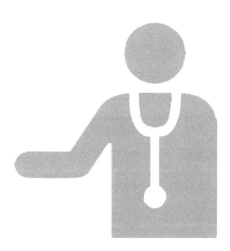

26. 수술이나 시술 받은 외래환자에게 주의사항 설명

(Going Home Instructions after Outpatient
Post−Procedure or Minor Surgery)

1. You have just had a surgical procedure.

   방금 수술(시술)을 받으셨습니다.

2. You could be drowsy for a couple of hours after your

   injection because of the sedative you may received.

   진정제를 투여 받아 몇 시간 동안 어지러울 수 있습니다.

3. You have no pain during one hour, because the area

   has been numbed with local anesthesia.

   한 시간 동안 국소마취 때문에 통증이 없습니다.

4. On the day of operation, you can expect some pain.

   수술 당일은 조금 아플 수 있습니다.

5. Take the prescribed medication if you have a pain attack.

   통증이 생기면 처방해 준 약을 드세요.

6. Fill the prescription at the pharmacy.

   약국에서 약을 사세요.

7. Don't change the dosage of medication.

   약 용량을 바꾸지 마세요.

8. If you see blood coming through the bandage,

   don't be alarmed.

   밴드 사이로 피가 나와도 놀라지는 마십시오.

9. Elevate your wound site and wrap some toweling around
   the bandage.

   상처부위를 높게 하고 붕대 주변에 수건으로 감아주세요.

10. Keep the site elevated and notify the doctor if bleeding
    continues.

    상처 부위를 높이 해도 피가 계속 나면 의사에게 알려주세요.

11. Don't remove suture and bandage.

    봉합사나 붕대를 풀지 마세요.

12. Watch for redness, swelling, persistent bleeding,
    and increased pain.

    빨개지거나, 붓고, 출혈이 있고, 통증이 심해지는 지 지켜보세요.

13. Keep the bandage clean and intact until your next visit.

    붕대를 다음 내원할 때까지 깨끗하게 유지하세요.

14. Don't drink alcohol beverages or smoke.

    술을 먹거나 담배를 피우시면 안 됩니다.

15. Immediately after discharge, you are go directly home
    and limit your activity.

    퇴원 후 바로 집으로 가고 활동을 하지 말아야 합니다.

16. If you received exercises from your doctor,
    start them as soon as possible.

    의사선생님이 바로 활동이 가능하다면 바로 시작하셔도 됩니다.

17. If you have severe pain, it is advisable to use ice
    at the operation site for 20 minutes of every hour.

    통증이 아주 심하면 시간당 20분 동안 얼음찜질을 해 주세요.

18. The medicine which was used to put the patient to sleep
    will be acting in the body for the next 24 hours,
    so you might get a little sleepy, you should not drive a car.
    진정제는 24시간 동안 몸에 작용을 하므로 졸릴 수 있으니
    운전을 하면 안 됩니다.

19. Your family or friend have to escort you to your home.
    당신 가족이나 친구가 반드시 집까지 데려다 주어야 합니다.

20. We suggest that a responsible adult be with the patient
    for the rest of the day.
    책임질 수 있는 성인이 하루를 함께 해주길 권합니다.

Conversation

N : You are going to have an operation.

수술을 받으시는군요.

I can see you worried.

걱정이 되시나 보군요.

P : Is it going to hurt?

아플까요?

N : Doctor will give you a local anesthetic.

의사선생님이 국소마취를 하실 것입니다.

It won't hurt much.

많이 아프지는 않을 것입니다.

P : That's a relief.

다행이네요.

N : The effect of the anesthetic will wear off in an hour.

한 시간 후면 마취가 풀립니다.

P : OK.

알겠습니다.

N : You'll need to sign a consent form.

서약서에 사인이 필요합니다.

Doctor will explain it in more detail.

의사 선생님이 더 자세히 설명해 주실 것입니다.

Have you got a family member here?

여기에 가족 어느 분이 게시나요?

P : Yes. My younger brother is here.

네 동생이 이곳에 있습니다.

He must be around.

주변에 있을 것입니다.

N : All finished.

모두 끝났습니다.

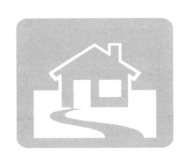

Your next appointment is －.

다음 예약 날짜는 －입니다.

If you have any question, call doctor －.

의문점이 있으면 －으로 의사에게 전화주세요.

If you have an emergency, you may call －.

만약 응급상황이면 － 로 전화주세요.

27. 호흡기 내과 질문들

Do you have a cough?

기침이 있나요?

Do you have a fever?

열이 있으세요?

Do you have a sore throat?

목이 아프세요?

Do you have a cough, sneezing or runny nose?

기침이나 콧물이 나오지는 않으세요?

How long have you had a cough?

기침이 얼마나 오래 되었죠?

When did your cough begin?

언제 기침이 시작되었죠?

When does the cough occur?

언제 기침이 나오지요?

Do you cough quite often?

자주 기침을 하시나요?

Do you get discomfort in your chest?

가슴이 불편하십니까?

Do you get any pain on breathing?

숨을 쉴 때 아프지는 않나요?

Do you get a pain in your chest when you cough?

기침을 할 때 가슴이 아프나요?

Have you had a cold recently?

최근에 감기에 걸린 적이 있나요?

Do you cough up phlegm?

가래가 나오나요?

How much do you bring up phlegm?

얼마나 가래가 많이 나오지요?

When do you bring up phlegm?

언제 가래가 나오지요?

What color is it?

색깔은 어떻지요?

Are you coughing up thick yellow or red phlegm ?

기침에서 노랗거나 붉은 가래가 나오지는 않던가요?

Are you coughing up blood?

기침에 피가 나오지는 않던가요?

Have you ever coughed up blood or bloody sputum?

피가 섞인 가래를 뱉은 적이 있나요?

Do you have a fever with the shortness of breath?

숨쉬기 힘이 들면서 열은 없나요?

Do you feel muscle aches or headaches?

근육통이나 두통은 없나요?

제 2 부

167

Does any position make it worse?

어떤 자세가 기침을 악화시키나요?

Do you have any difficulty with your breathing?

숨을 쉬는데 불편하지는 않나요?

Do you get short of breath?

숨이 가쁘시나요?

Are you troubled by short of breath?

숨이 가빠 힘들지는 않나요?

Have you ever had any shortness of breath?

숨쉬기 곤란한 적이 있었나요?

Is it more difficult to breathe in or breathe out?

숨을 들이키거나 내쉴 때 언제가 더 힘이 들죠?

Does it hurt when you breathe?

숨을 쉴 때 아픈가요?

Have you ever had asthma or allergy?

천식이나 알러지를 앓은 적이 있나요?

Are you using a puffer for your asthma?

천식으로 분무기를 사용하나요?

Do you have an inhaler for your asthma?

천식을 위한 분무기를 가지고 있나요?

How many puffs do you use per day?

하루에 몇 번 불죠?

Have you ever suffered from tuberculosis?

결핵에 걸린 적은 없습니까?

When was the last time you had a tuberculosis test?

결핵 검사를 마지막으로 한 때가 어디죠?

Does anyone else in your family have this cough?

당신 가족 중에 이런 기침을 하는 사람이 있습니까?

Do you have a headache or general aches?

두통이나 몸이 아프지는 않나요?

Do you have a fever or chill?

열이 나거나 오한이 있나요?

제 2 부

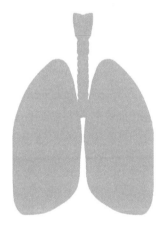

28. 심장 내과 질문들

Do you know the fact that you have hypertension?

당신이 고혈압을 가지고 있다는 사실을 알고 있나요?

When did you know that?

언제 그것을 알았죠?

Do you have a history of hypertension in your family?

가족 중에 고혈압이 있었던 적이 있나요?

Do you check your blood pressure regularly?

당신의 혈압을 규칙적으로 측정하고 있습니까?

Do you ever have palpitations?

가슴이 두근거린 적은 없나요?

Do you have any chest discomfort or chest pain?

가슴이 답답하거나 아프지는 않나요?

Do you have shortness of breath?

숨이 차지는 않습니까?

Do you get pain in your chest?

가슴이 아픕니까?

Do you feel chest discomfort?

가슴이 불편합니까?

Have you ever had heart problems?

심장에 문제가 있었던 적이 있었나요?

Do you have pressure or tightness in your chest?

가슴이 묵직하거나 답답하지는 않나요?

Have you ever felt your heart fluttering very quickly?

심장이 아주 두근거린 적이 없나요?

Does the pain move around and spread anywhere?

통증이 주위로 퍼져가나요?

Do you feel any discomfort in other area?

다른 곳에 불편감은 없나요?

Do you have any episode of pressure under the chest
 by cold air or activity?

찬 공기나 운동 후 가슴 아래에 통증이 있었던 적이 있나요?

Tell me about your chest pain and how it began?

가슴 통증과 그것이 어떻게 시작되었는지 말씀해 주실래요?

Does the pain occur commonly when you are exercising?

운동할 때 통증이 잘 일어나던가요?

How do you feel your pain?

통증의 느낌이 어떤가요?

Could you describe the character of the pain?

통증이 어떤지 설명해 주실래요?

What about breathing when you have the pain?

통증이 있을 때 숨 쉬는 것은 어떠했나요?

Do you have episodes of shortness of breath?

숨이 가쁜 적은 없었나요?

Are you troubled by shortness of breath?

숨이 차지는 않습니까?

Have you ever fainted?

졸도한 적은 있나요?

Have you ever had rheumatic fever?

류마티스열을 앓은 적은 없습니까?

Did you ever have an electrocardiogram?

심전도 검사를 받은 적이 있습니까?

Have you recently had an echocardiogram?

최근에 심장 초음파 검사를 하셨나요?

Do you feel dizzy?

어지러움을 느끼나요?

Do you suffer from any other problems?

다른 문제는 없나요?

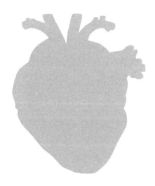

29. 내분비 내과 질문들

Do you have diabetes?

당뇨병이 있나요?

When did you get it?

언제 당뇨병에 걸렸죠?

Do you have a history of diabetes in the family?

가족 중에 당뇨병이 있었던 적이 있나요?

Are you checking your blood sugar regularly?

혈당을 규칙적으로 체크하고 있습니까?

Do you check blood sugar today?

오늘 혈당을 측정하였나요?

What are your sugars in the morning?

아침에 혈당이 얼마였죠?

Are you taking any tablet or insulin?

약을 먹거나 인슐린을 맞고 있나요?

Are you taking your pills for your sugar?

혈당 조절을 위해 약을 복용하고 있나요?

Do you take insulin?

인슐린을 맞고 있나요?

Have you been adjusting your insulin?

인슐린을 조절하고 있나요?

Have you been adjusting insulin when it goes high?

혈당이 높으면 인슐린을 조절하나요?

Do you do anything when you have low sugars?

혈당이 낮을 때 어떻게 조치하시죠?

Do you have any tingling of the hands or feet?

손이나 발이 저리시지는 않습니까?

Do you feel thirst or fatigue?

갈증이나 피곤함을 느끼십니까?

Have you been drinking excessive fluids?

물을 많이 마시나요?

Are you trying to lose some weight?

체중을 줄이려고 노력하고 있나요?

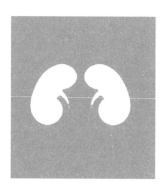

30. 소화기 내과 질문들

Do you have abdominal discomfort?

배가 불편하시나요?

Do you get pain in your abdomen?

배가 아프시나요?

Do you have gastric pain?

위가 아프시나요?

Where does your belly hurt you?

배 어느 부위가 아프죠?

Do you have right lower quadrant abdominal discomfort
 or pain ?

배 오른쪽 아래가 아프거나 불편한가요?

What kind of discomfort?

어떤 종류의 불편함이죠?

Do you feel abdominal tenderness?

배를 누르면 아픈가요?

What kind of pain?

어떤 종류의 통증이죠?

What do you feel like?

어떻게 느끼시는데요?

How often do you get pain?

통증이 얼마나 자주 발생하죠?

Do you feel pain after meal?

식사 후 통증이 오나요?

Do certain foods bring on pain?

어떤 음식이 통증을 일으키나요?

Do you feel pain before meal?

식사 전에 통증이 오나요?

If you eat, do you feel better?

만약 먹으면 좋아지던가요?

How soon after eating?

먹고 얼마 후 그렇던가요?

Do you feel nausea or vomiting?

오심이나 구토를 느끼나요?

Are you gonna throw up?

토할 것 같나요?

How much do you vomit?

얼마나 많이 토했죠?

How often do you vomit?

얼마나 자주 토했죠?

When do you vomit?

언제 토했죠?

Have you noticed any blood in your vomit?

토할 때 피 같은 것은 못 보셨나요?

What color is the vomit?

토한 것들의 색깔이 어떠했습니까?

Do you bring up acid?

신물이 넘어 오나요?

How about your digestion?

소화는 어떻습니까?

Did you have any other symptoms with your stomach pain?

위통과 함께 다른 증상은 없었나요?

Have you ever diagnosed with stomach ulcer?

위궤양이라고 진단 받은 적이 있나요?

How are the bowel movements?

화장실 가는 것은 어떻습니까?

Are the bowels all right?

화장실 가는 것은 괜찮나요?

Do you have any problem moving your bowels?

대변보는 것에 문제가 있나요?

Do you have constipation?

변비가 있나요?

Difficult bowel movement?

대변을 보기가 어렵나요?

Painful bowel movement?

아프나요?

Absent bowel movement?

변비인가요?

Infrequent bowel movement?

불규칙한가요?

Do you have pain with your bowel movements?

대변을 볼 때 배가 아프나요?

Do you have discomfort while moving your bowel?

대변 눌 때 배가 불편하나요?

How many times did you have bowel movements today?

오늘 대변을 몇 번 보셨지요?

How often do you have bowel movements?

얼마나 자주 대변을 보시죠?

Do you have fewer than three bowel movements each week?

일주일에 3번보다 적게 대변을 보십니까?

Do you often have a hard time passing stools?

대변을 보기 힘들 때가 있습니까?

Have you had chronic constipation?

만성적인 변비를 가지고 있나요?

Do you take laxative?

변비약을 먹었나요?

Do you get pain during passing your motions?

대변볼 때 통증이 있나요?

Do you have diarrhea?

설사는 하지 않나요?

Since when have you had diarrhea?

언제부터 설사가 있었죠?

How often did you have diarrhea?

설사를 몇 번이나 했죠?

Does any particular food upset you?

배탈을 나게 한 어떤 특별한 음식이 있었나요?

Have you eaten a food that might be spoiled?

상한 음식을 먹지는 않았나요?

Do you have dry feces or hard feces?

대변이 마르고 딱딱하지는 않나요?

Have you noticed any changes in your urine or stool?

소변이나 대변에 어떤 이상은 없나요?

Have you ever passed any bloody stool?

혈변을 눈 적은 없나요?

Have you ever passed any black stool?

검은 변을 눈 적은 없나요?

What about color of stool?

대변이 무슨 색이죠?

Have you noticed an abnormal smell?

이상한 냄새는 나지 않던가요?

Do you suffer from loss of appetite?

식욕이 없나요?

Do you feel abdominal swelling or bloating?

복부 팽만감이나 가스 찬 것을 느낍니까?

Have you lost your weight?

몸무게가 줄었나요?

Have you traveled recently to another country?

최근에 다른 나라로 여행을 갔다 오지 않았나요?

Are you presently taking an antibiotics or other medicine?

최근에 항생제나 다른 약을 복용하지는 않았나요?

Do you have itching around your anus?

항문 주변으로 가렵지는 않나요?

Have you recently had an ultrasound scan of your abdomen?

최근에 복부 초음파 검사를 하셨나요?

Do you feel fatigue?

피곤함을 느낍니까?

Do you experience unexplained weight loss?

이유 없이 체중이 감소하나요?

Do you experience loss of appetite?

식욕이 없나요?

Did you ever have jaundice?

황달이 있었던 적이 있나요?

Did you have any other symptoms with your jaundice?

황달 외에 다른 증상은 없었나요?

Do you feel itching sensation?

가렵지는 않나요?

Did you have vaccine against hepatitis B.

B형 간염 예방 주사를 맞았나요?

31. 일반 외과 질문들

Do you have abdominal discomfort?

배가 불편한가요?

Do you get pain in your abdomen?

배가 아픕니까?

Where does your belly hurt you?

배 어느 부위가 아프죠?

Where does your abdomen hurt the most?

배 어느 부위가 가장 아프죠?

Do you feel abdominal pain when I touch?

배를 누르면 아픈가요?

How often do you get pain?

통증이 얼마나 자주 발생하죠.

Do you have any abdominal palpable mass?

복부에 만져지는 혹은 없나요?

Have you ever passed any bloody stool?

혈변을 눈 적은 없나요?

Have you ever passed any black stool?

검은 변을 눈 적은 없나요?

Do you feel nausea or vomiting?

오심이나 구토를 느끼나요?

Have you ever had any injuries?

다친 적은 없나요?

Have you had any masses in your breasts?

유방에 혹이 있나요?

When did you first notice this lump?

언제 이 혹을 처음 발견하셨죠?

Did you experience any pain in your breast?

유방이 아픈 적이 있나요?

Do your breasts get sore before your period?

생리 전에 유방이 아픈가요?

Have you ever tried examining your breasts?

유방을 검사 해 본 적이 있나요?

Do you feel swelling in your neck?

목이 부은 것을 느끼나요?

Have you had any thyroid trouble?

갑상선에 문제가 있었던 적이 있나요?

Have you ever noticed any enlargement of lymph nodes?

임파선이 부은 적은 없었나요?

Have you noticed any lumps anywhere in your body?

몸에 혹 같은 것은 없나요?

Have you ever had a hernia?

탈장 같은 것은 없었나요?

Did you ever have jaundice?

황달이 있었던 적이 있나요?

Have you lost any weight?

몸무게가 줄었나요?

Have you ever notices any edema in your legs?

다리가 부은 적이 없나요?

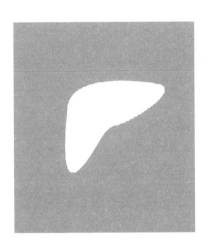

32. 산부인과 질문들

Do you have regular periods?

생리는 규칙적인가요?

Are your periods irregular?

생리가 불규칙적인가요?

Are you on your period?

생리중인가요?

Are you missing your period?

생리를 걸렀나요?

When was the period before that?

그 전의 생리는 언제였지요?

When did your period start?

언제 생리가 시작되었죠?

When was your last period?

마지막 생리가 언제였죠?

Do you still see your periods?

아직도 생리중인가요?

Have you stopped having periods?

생리가 멈추었나요?

Do you get hot flushes?

얼굴이 화끈거린 적이 있나요?

Have your periods always been regular in the past?

과거에 생리는 항상 규칙적이었나요?

When was your first period?

언제 생리가 처음 시작했죠?

How do you feel before your periods start?

생리 전 어떻게 느끼죠?

How long do you have periods?

생리가 얼마나 지속되죠?

How many days have you been bleeding?

얼마 동안 출혈이 있었죠?

Are your periods heavy?

생리가 많나요?

How much do you bleed?

얼마나 나오죠?

Do you have much flow each time?

항상 양이 많나요?

How many pads do you use each day?

매일 생리대를 얼마나 쓰죠?

Do you use pads as well as tampons?

생리대와 탐폰을 같이 쓰나요?

Do you have menstrual cramp?

생리통이 있나요?

Where does your belly hurt you?

배 어느 부위가 아프죠?

Do you get pain in your lower abdomen?

아랫배가 아픕니까?

Have your periods become more painful?

생리 중 점점 더 아프던가요?

When was your last cervical smear?

자궁경부 검사를 마지막으로 한 적이 언제죠?

Have you had regular cervical smears?

정기적으로 자궁경부 검사를 하나요?

Do you have vaginal discharge?

질 분비가 있나요?

Do you have vaginal bleeding without menstruation?

생리도 없이 출혈이 있나요?

How long have you had this discharge?

얼마나 오래 이 분비가 있었죠?

How often do you get it?

얼마나 자주 있죠?

How much is there?

얼마나 많나요?

What color is it?

색깔은 어떻죠?

Do you have any itching sensation?

간지러운가요?

Have you ever been pregnant?

임신한 적은 있나요?

When did you have sex last?

최근에 섹스는 언제 하셨죠?

Do you use an intra-uterine device(IUD)?

자궁 내 피임기구는 쓰지 않습니까?

Do you take any contraception?

피임약을 먹고 있습니까?

Have you ever had any abortion?

유산한 적이 있었나요?

Have you ever had a D&C?

인공중절수술을 받은 적이 있었나요?

Why did you have a D & C?

왜 인공중절수술을 받았죠?

Do you have any history of ectopic pregnancy?

자궁 외 임신을 한 적이 있나요?

Do you have missed periods?

월경을 지나쳤나요?

How long has it been since your last period?

마지막 생리 후 얼마나 되었죠?

제 2 부

Could you be pregnant?

임신 가능성이 있나요?

When was your last period?

마지막 생리가 언제였죠?

Have you had sexual intercourse?

섹스를 하였나요?

When was your last contact?

마지막 섹스가 언제였죠?

Have you taken a pregnancy test?

임신 검사를 해 보셨나요?

Are you pregnant?

임신하셨나요?

How far along?

얼마나 되었죠?

How long have you been pregnant?

임신한 지 얼마나 되었죠?

When is your due date?

언제가 분만일이죠?

Do you have morning sickness?

입덧을 하나요?

Do you have swelling and tenderness over the breast?

유방 위가 붓고 아픈가요?

Is this your first pregnancy?

초산인가요?

Have you ever been pregnant?

임신 한 적이 있나요?

How many times have you been pregnant?

몇 번 임신을 하셨죠?

Have you been pregnant two times?

2번째 임신하셨나요?

When was the date of your last delivery?

마지막 분만이 언제였죠?

Did you have any trouble during pregnancy?

임신 중 이상은 없었나요?

Have you had any cramps or bleeding?

배가 아프거나 출혈한 적이 있나요?

Have you ever had any spontaneous abortion(miscarriage)?

자연유산이 있었나요?

Have you ever had a C-sec?

제왕 절개술을 받은 적이 있나요?

Did you have preeclampsia before?

전에 임신 자간증에 걸린 적이 있나요?

When did the contraction start?

언제 진통이 시작되었죠?

Can you feel the baby move?

아기가 움직이는 것을 느끼나요?

Are you having contractions?

자궁 수축이 있나요?

How frequent are the contractions?

자궁 수축이 얼마나 자주 있죠?

Did you have a normal delivery?

정상적인 분만이었나요?

Was your child delivered by C—section?

아기가 제왕절개술로 태어났나요?

How long were you in labor?

분만 시간이 얼마였죠?

Did you have any complications when you had delivery?

분만 중 어떤 부작용은 없었나요?

33. 소아 청소년과 질문들

How old is your baby?

아기가 몇 살이죠?

How much does your baby weigh?

아기의 몸무게가 얼마죠?

Does your baby have a fever?

아기가 열이 있나요?

Did your baby vomit?

아기가 토하던가요?

Did your baby have fits?

아기가 발작을 했나요?

When did your baby start having fits?

언제 발작을 시작했죠?

Does your baby have cold symptoms?

아기에게 감기 증상이 있나요?

Does your baby seem to have diarrhea?

아기가 설사를 하는 것 같던가요?

Is the bowel movement mostly yellow?

변이 전부 노랗던가요?

Does your baby have hard bowel movements?

아기가 대변을 잘 누지 못하나요?

Does your baby cry before bowel movements?

변을 보기 전에 울던가요?

How old is your child?

아이가 몇 살이죠?

Has your child been vaccinated as scheduled?

아이가 스케줄대로 예방 접종을 받았나요?

Can you recall about your child's immunization?

아이의 예방 접종에 대해 기억이 나나요?

Did you have any problems with pregnancy or birth?

임신 중 또는 분만 중 어떤 문제는 없었나요?

Has your child had any surgery or hospitalization?

아이가 수술을 받거나 입원한 적이 있나요?

Is there any mass or lump on your baby?

아이에게 혹이나 멍울이 없던가요?

Is there any change in behavior?

행동에 어떤 변화가 있던가요?

Does your child have earache or sore throat?

아이가 귀가 아프다거나 목이 아프다고 하지는 않던가요?

I will check the temperature.

체온을 측정하겠습니다.

Would you take off your shoes and stand on the scales?

신발을 벗고 체중계에 서 줄래?

Could you come and stand over here to check your height?

키를 측정하게 이곳으로 와서 서줄래?

How many children do you have?

아이들이 몇 명이나 있죠?

How old are they?

아이들이 몇 살이죠?

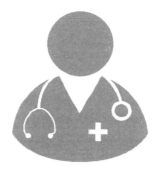

34. 정형외과 질문들

Where is your pain?

어디가 아프시죠?

Did you get hurt?

다쳤나요?

How did you get hurt?

어떻게 다쳤어요?

Did you fall down?

넘어졌나요?

Did you get hit (beaten)?

맞았나요?

Did you get in an accident?

사고가 났나요?

When did accident happen?

언제 일어난 것이죠?

Do you feel any pain here?

여기가 아픈가요?

Does your neck hurt?

목이 아프나요?

Does your back hurt?

허리가 아프나요?

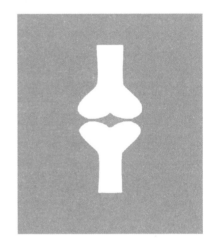

Does the pain come with motion?

움직이면 아프나요?

Where in your body does it hurt?

몸 어느 부분이 아프나요?

Do you get pain in your joints?

관절이 아프나요?

Do you get pain in your muscles?

근육이 아프나요?

How long have you had it?

얼마나 오랫동안 아팠어요?

How frequently do you have pain?

얼마나 자주 통증이 발생하죠?

Do you have redness or swelling?

붉거나 부종이 있나요?

Which joints have a problem?

어떤 관절들이 아프시죠?

Do you have any swelling in your joints?

당신의 관절에서 부은 곳은 없나요?

Do you have any pain or stiffness in any joint?

관절이 아프거나 굳어지는 곳은 없나요?

Do the joints feel stiff?

관절들이 굳어지는 느낌이 있나요?

Is the pain worse in the morning?

아침에 통증이 더 심해지던가요?

How long does the stiffness last?

굳어지는 느낌이 얼마나 되었죠?

Does the pain stay in one region?

통증이 한 곳에만 머무릅니까?

Are one or more joints swollen and tender?

하나 또는 여러 개의 관절이 붓거나 아프지는 않나요?

When did you get these multiple joint pains?

언제부터 이러한 다발성 관절통이 있으셨죠?

How about when you walk or exercise?

걷거나 운동할 때는 어떻습니까?

Have you ever had fracture of bones?

골절이 있었던 적은 없습니까?

Have you ever had rheumatoid arthritis?

류마티스 관절염을 앓았던 적은 없습니까?

Did the pain come from a repeated motion?

통증이 자주 움직여서 오던가요?

Does the movement make the pain more severe?

움직이면 통증이 더 심하던가요?

Do you have back pain with leg pain?

다리와 함께 허리가 아픈가요?

Do you have tingling sensation in your arms or legs?

팔이나 다리가 저리지는 않나요?

Do you have any radiating pain in your arms or legs?

팔이나 다리에 방사통은 없습니까?

196

Do you have any weakness in your arms or legs?

팔이나 다리가 약하지는 않나요?

Can you feel me touching them?

제가 만지는 것을 느끼시나요?

Wiggle your fingers and toes.

손가락, 발가락을 움직여 보세요.

Squeeze my hand.

제 손을 쥐어보세요.

Push down with your toes on my hand like a gas pedal.

차 페달 밟듯이 발가락으로 제 손을 눌러 보세요.

Bend your elbows and knees.

팔꿈치와 무릎을 구부려 보세요.

Pull your arms.

팔을 당겨 보세요.

Do you have a history of knee joint locking?

무릎이 굽혔다가 펴지지 않은 경우가 있었나요?

Are you being worked too hard in your job or exercise?

당신은 지금 혹시 무리한 일이나 운동을 하고 있습니까?

Do you have any history of falling or trauma?

넘어지거나 다친 적이 있습니까?

If you go out into the cold, do your fingers change color and

become painful?

만약 찬 곳으로 나가면, 손가락 색이 변하고 아프기 시작하나요?

제 2 부

197

35. 신경외과 질문들

Do you have headaches?

머리가 아픕니까?

Where in your head does it hurt?

머리 어디가 아프시죠?

Which part hurts the most?

어느 부분이 가장 아프지요?

How did you get hurt?

어떻게 다쳤죠?

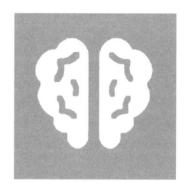

Did you hurt your head?

머리를 다쳤나요?

Did you fall (slip, trip)?

넘어졌나요?

Did you hit your head?

머리를 부딪쳤나요?

How far did you fall?

얼마나 높은 곳에서 떨어졌지요?

Do you get pain in your head?

머리가 아프나요?

Do you have frequent headaches?

머리가 자주 아프나요?

Are you dizzy?

어지러운가요?

Do you ever feel sick?

메스꺼운 적이 있나요?

Did you lose your consciousness?

의식을 잃었었습니까?

Have you had any nausea or vomiting?

오심이나 구토를 하였나요?

Have you ever had a head injury before?

전에 머리를 다친 적이 있나요?

Have you ever had any dizziness?

어지러웠던 적은 없나요?

Do you remember when you had an accident?

사고가 났을 때가 기억나나요?

Have you injured your head or been knocked out recently?

최근에 머리를 다치거나 맞은 적이 있나요?

Did you suffer from headaches?

두통이 있었나요?

When was the first time you had headaches?

두통을 느낀 처음이 언제죠?

Do you have any history of fainting suddenly?

갑자기 기절했던 적은 없었나요?

Are you dizzy when you stand up?

일어날 때 어지러운가요?

When do you feel dizziness?

언제 어지러움을 느끼죠?

How long does the dizziness last?

어지러움이 얼마나 지속되죠?

How often do you have dizziness?

얼마나 자주 어지러움을 느끼나요?

How long do the headaches last?

두통이 얼마나 지속되죠?

Have you ever had this kind of headache in the past?

과거에도 이런 종류의 두통이 있었습니까?

Do you have a history of high blood pressure?

고혈압 경력은 있나요?

Do you have pressure around your eyes?

눈 주위에 압박감 등은 없습니까?

Are there worse in the morning or evening?

아침이나 저녁에 악화되나요?

What kind of medicine do you take to relieve your headaches?

두통을 없애기 위해 무슨 약을 먹었죠?

When did the seizure start?

언제부터 경련을 했죠?

Have you ever had the seizure in the past?

과거에 경련을 한 적이 있나요?

How often do you have the seizure?

얼마나 자주 경련을 하죠?

What triggered the seizure?

어떤 것이 경련을 일으키죠?

Do you have stiff neck?

목이 뻣뻣하지는 않으세요?

Do you have any problems with your hearing and seeing?

듣거나 보는데 문제가 있나요?

Have you been having any problems with your memory?

기억에 문제가 있지는 않나요?

Can you feel me touching here?

제가 만지는 곳을 느끼시나요?

Have you noticed any numbness, tingling or weakness
in your limbs?

팔 다리가 감각이 없거나 저리거나 약하지는 않나요?

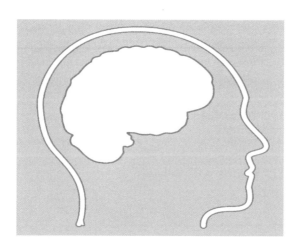

36. 안과 질문들

Do you have any problems with your eyes?

눈에 문제가 있나요?

Do you get any kind of problems with your eyes?

당신의 눈에 이상이 있습니까?

Do you have eye pain?

눈이 아프나요?

Do you have blurred vision?

눈이 흐린가요?

Do you have vision change?

시력의 변화가 있나요?

Have you noticed any change in your vision?

시력에 변화가 있나요?

When did this problem begin?

언제 이 문제가 생겼죠?

Both eyes? one eye?

두 눈 모두인가요? 한 눈인가요?

Have you ever worn glasses?

안경을 쓴 적이 있나요?

Can you see very well without glasses?

안경도 없이 잘 볼 수 있나요?

Can you see clearly both far away and close up?

먼 곳이나 가까운 곳을 명료하게 볼 수 있나요?

Are you near-sighted (myopia)?

근시인가요?

Are you far-sighted (hyperopia)?

원시인가요?

Do you have difficulty reading the book?

책을 읽기 힘든가요?

How long have you been wearing glasses?

얼마나 오랫동안 안경을 썼지요?

When did you wear them?

언제 안경을 썼지요?

What were they for?

무엇을 교정하려고 안경을 썼지요?

Are they for distance, near, or both?

안경은 원시? 근시? 혹은 난시를 위한 건가요?

Do you wear contact lens?

콘택트 렌즈를 끼나요?

How often do you replace them?

얼마나 자주 갈아 끼우죠?

What other symptoms do you experience with this problem?

이 문제와 함께 다른 증상들도 있나요?

Have you ever had any medical attention to your eyes?

당신의 눈에 대해 의학적으로 주의를 받은 적이 있나요?

Did you have any surgery, injuries, or serious infections?

어떤 수술이나 상처나 감염된 적이 있나요?

Did you have any inflammation in your eyelids?

안검에 염증이 있었나요?

Have you ever had any eye inflammation?

눈에 염증이 있었던 적은 없나요?

Have you ever worn an eye patch?

아이 패치를 쓴 적이 있나요?

Have you ever used any medication for your eyes?

당신의 눈을 위해 약을 쓴 적이 있나요?

Do you take any eye drops?

안약을 썼나요?

Have you ever been told that you have cataracts, glaucoma,
or any other eye disease?

백내장, 녹내장, 또는 다른 눈 질환이 있다고 들은 적이 있나요?

Have you ever had any eye injuries?

눈을 다친 적이 있나요?

Do you have symptoms of presbyopia?

노안증상을 느끼고 있나요?

37. 이비인후과 질문들

Do you have good hearing?

잘 들리나요?

Do you have hearing loss?

귀가 잘 안 들리나요?

Do you have hearing loss in one or both ears?

한쪽 또는 양쪽에서 귀가 잘 안 들리나요?

Can you hear well what others say?

다른 사람들이 말할 때 잘 들리나요?

Are you working around loud noises?

일할 때 소음에 계속 노출되나요?

Has your hearing loss occurred gradually as you have aged?

나이가 들면서 점차 귀가 안 들리던가요?

Do you wear a hearing aid?

보청기를 사용하시나요?

Do you have ear pain?

귀가 아프나요?

Do you have ear discharge?

귀에서 진물이 나오나요?

Do you have a pain deep in the ear?

귀 안쪽 깊은 곳이 아프나요?

Do you have thick drainage from the ear canal?

귀에서 진한 분비물이 나오나요?

Is the pus woozing from your ears?

귀에서 고름이 나오나요?

Do you have pain behind your ear?

귀 뒤쪽이 아프나요?

Do you have tenderness when you touch the bone behind ear?

귀 뒤의 뼈를 만지면 아프나요?

Does your ear hurt when I pull on the ear?

귀를 잡아당기면 아프나요?

How often does ear pain occur?

귀 통증이 얼마나 자주 발생하죠?

Do you hear strange sounds?

이상한 소리들이 들리나요?

What does it sound like?

어떤 소음이 들리나요?

Do you hear fluid in your ear?

귀 안에서 물 흐르는 소리가 느껴지나요?

Do you feel water in your ear?

귀에 물 있는 게 느껴지나요?

Do you have ringing in your ears?

귀울림이 있나요?

Have you experienced any ringing in your ears?

귀울림을 경험한 적이 있나요?

Do you have a ringing in one or both ears?

귀울림이 한쪽 또는 양쪽에서 있나요?

Which ear is worse?

어느 쪽이 더 나쁘죠?

Do you feel pressure that can't be cleared with swallowing?

삼켜도 좋아지지 않는 귀 안의 압박감 같은 것이 있나요?

Do you have bouts of dizziness?

갑자기 어지러운 적이 있나요?

Do you feel dizziness?

어지럽나요?

Do you have a cough or runny nose?

기침을 하거나 콧물이 나나요?

Do you have sore throat?

목이 아프나요?

Do you have lumps or swelling in the throat?

목안에 혹이 있거나 부었나요?

Do you have any difficulty swallowing?

삼키기 힘드나요?

Do you get sore throat quite often?

목안이 자주 아프나요?

How often do you get sore throat?

얼마나 자주 목이 아프죠?

Have you had your tonsils out?

편도선을 제거하셨나요?

Have you ever had any ulcer in your mouth or on your lips?

입안이나 입술에 궤양이 생긴 적은 없나요?

Have you noticed any changes in your voice?

당신의 목소리가 변했나요?

Do you have a fever or cold symptom?

열이나 감기 증상이 있나요?

Do you catch cold easily?

쉽게 감기에 잘 걸리나요?

Do you have frequent nosebleeds?

자주 코피가 나나요?

38. 피부과 질문들

Do you have any skin problems?

피부에 어떤 문제가 있나요?

Did you get a bug bite?

벌레에 물렸나요?

Did you get bitten by insect?

곤충에 물렸나요?

Do you have any rashes?

발진이 있나요?

When did the rash start?

언제 발진이 있었죠?

Did the rash spread?

발진이 퍼지던가요?

Do you feel itching?

가려운가요?

When does your skin feel itchy?

언제 피부가 가렵죠?

Where is it most severe?

어디가 가장 심하죠?

Do you have any eczema?

습진이 있나요?

Is there anything that aggravates your eczema?

습진을 악화시키는 것이 있나요?

What have you tried for your eczema?

습진치료를 위해 어떻게 하셨죠?

Do you have an atopic dermatitis?

아토피 피부염이 있나요?

Do you have atopic problems?

아토피 문제가 있나요?

Do you have any allergies?

알러지 병력이 있나요?

Do you have any history of any rash?

발진이 있었던 적이 있었나요?

Have you ever experienced any skin eruptions on your body?

몸에 피부 발진이 일어난 적이 있나요?

Are you on any medication?

어떤 약을 복용하고 있나요?

Did you eat something special?

특별한 음식을 먹었나요?

Does anyone in your family suffer from skin problem?

가족 중에 피부 문제를 가지고 있는 사람이 있나요?

Is your skin dry?

피부가 건조하나요?

Do you get any spots?

점들이 있나요?

39. 비뇨기과 질문들

How about your urination?

소변보는 것은 어떤가요?

Do you have any problems passing water?

소변을 보는데 문제가 있나요?

Do you have any difficulties in voiding your urine?

소변을 보는데 힘이 드나요?

Do you feel like urinating often?

소변을 자주 보고 싶나요?

Do you have problems starting the urine stream?

소변을 보는데 처음에 어려움이 있나요?

Do you have a weak urinary stream?

소변이 약하나요?

Do you dribble urine after you urinate?

소변을 본 다음에도 소변이 뚝뚝 떨어지나요?

Do you wake many times at night to urinate?

소변을 보기 위해 밤에 자주 일어나나요?

Did you see blood in your urine?

소변에서 피를 보았나요?

Is your urine cloudy?

소변이 탁하나요?

Where does your belly hurt you?

배 어느 부위가 아프죠?

Do you have any pain in your abdomen, side or back?

배나 옆구리, 허리가 아프지는 않나요?

Do you get pain in your side?

옆구리가 아픕니까?

Do you have a fever and flank pain?

열이 나고 옆구리가 아프나요?

Do you have any history of renal stone?

신장 결석에 걸린 적이 있나요?

Did you ever have ureteral stone?

요관 결석에 걸린 적이 없나요?

Do you have pain into the groin?

서혜부 안쪽이 아프나요?

Is there pain behind the scrotum?

음낭 뒤쪽으로 통증이 있나요?

Have you ever had a kidney or bladder infection?

신장염이나 방광염을 앓은 적이 있습니까?

Do you feel pain in your bladder?

방광이 아프나요?

Do you have any pain or burning while urinating?

소변을 눌 때 아프거나 화끈거리나요?

Do you have pain in your penis when you urinate?

소변을 볼 때 음경이 아프나요?

Do you have a discharge from the tip of the penis?

물건 끝부분에서 뭐가 나오나요?

Did you see pus in your urine?

소변에서 고름을 보았나요?

Have you ever had any veneral diseases?

성병에 걸린 적이 있나요?

Do you leak when you cough?

기침을 하면 소변을 흘리나요?

When do you have leakage?

언제 요실금이 있죠?

How many pads do you use per day?

하루에 몇 개의 패드를 쓰시죠?

Do you have a sensation of not emptying your bladder

completely after you have finished urinating?

소변을 다 눈 후에도 방광이 빈 것 같지 않은 느낌이 드나요?

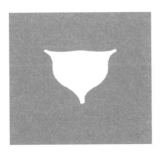

40. 치과 질문들

Do you have toothache?

치통이 있나요?

Which tooth is painful?

어느 치아가 아프죠?

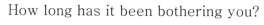

How long has it been bothering you?

언제부터 아프셨죠?

Do you feel pain in chewing?

씹을 때 아픈가요?

Do you have difficulty in chewing?

씹기가 힘드나요?

Do you have pain when you eat?

먹을 때 아프나요?

Do you feel pain when you drink cold water?

찬 물을 마실 때 아프나요?

Do you have tooth becoming loose?

흔들리는 치아가 있나요?

When did you have your teeth out?

언제 치아를 뽑았죠?

Do your gums bleed easily?

잇몸에서 쉽게 피가 나나요?

Do you have pain in your gums?

잇몸이 아픈가요?

Do you have any swelling in your gums?

잇몸이 부었나요?

How long have you had toothache?

얼마나 오랫동안 치통이 있었나요?

Do you have any discomfort with your mouth?

입안에 불편한 점이 있나요?

Do you have bad breath?

구취가 심하나요?

How often do you brush?

얼마나 자주 양치질을 하시죠?

Have you ever got dental treatment?

치과치료를 받은 적이 있나요?

Do you wear denture?

틀니를 사용하나요?

When did you start to use denture?

언제부터 틀니를 하셨죠?

41. 정신건강 의학과 질문들

How has your mood been lately?

최근 기분이 어떤가요?

How would you describe your mood now?

지금 기분이 어떠하시죠?

Would you tell me something about what's bothering you?

당신을 괴롭히는 것에 대해 말해줄래요?

Do you felt sad or depressed?

슬프거나 우울함을 느끼나요?

Do you have anything worry about?

무슨 걱정거리가 있나요?

What's your concern?

걱정거리가 무엇이죠?

Are you optimistic?

낙천주의자입니까?

Are you pessimistic?

염세주의자입니까?

Do you get angry more easily than usual?

보통 때 보다 더 자주 화를 내나요?

Do you feel life isn't worth living any more?

삶이 더 살 가치가 없다고 느끼나요?

216

Do emotional problems at work seem to make it worse?

직장에서의 감정이 증상을 더 나쁘게 만들던가요?

How have you been sleeping?

잠자는 것은 어떤가요?

Do you have any difficulty falling asleep?

잠드는 것에 문제가 있나요?

Are you able to sleep when you want to sleep?

잠자고 싶을 때 잠을 잘 수 있나요?

How long does it take you to fall asleep?

잠자려면 얼마나 시간이 걸리죠?

What is your usual bed time?

보통 몇 시에 자죠?

What time do you usually get up?

언제 보통 일어나죠?

Do you wake up early than usual?

보통보다 일찍 일어나나요?

What is your average total sleep time?

평균 수면시간이 얼마나 되죠?

Does anything interrupt your sleep?

수면을 어떤 것이 방해하나요?

How long have you had difficulty sleeping?

수면장애가 얼마나 오래되었죠?

Have you ever taken some medicine for sleep?

잠을 자기 위해서 약을 먹은 적이 있나요?

Are you very nervous?

아주 예민한 편인가요?

What stress do you experience in your relationship?

타인과의 관계에서 어떤 스트레스를 느끼나요?

Do you have any problems with your work?

일하는 데 어떤 문제가 있나요?

Do you enjoy your work?

일하는 것이 즐겁나요?

Do you have any problems controlling your emotions?

당신의 감정을 조절하는데 문제가 있나요?

Have you been having any problems with your memory?

기억에 문제가 있지는 않나요?

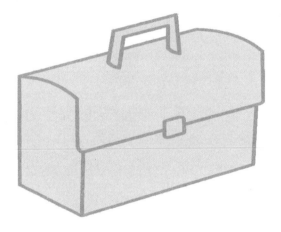

Everyday is another chance
to become the person we want to be.

Part III

Health Check Up, Radiology, Laboratory Room and Administration

제 3부

건강 검진, 방사선과, 임상병리과 및 원무과

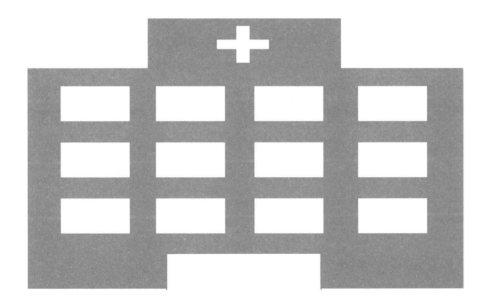

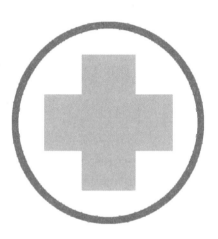

42. 정기 건강 검진
(Regular Medical Check Up)

1. Welcome to the health check up center.

   건강검진 센터에 오신 것을 환영합니다.

2. Have you ever visited hospital check up center?

   병원 건강검진 센터에 오신 적이 있으신가요?

3. Please have a seat.

   의자에 앉으세요.

4. Would you please fill out this form?

   이 양식을 작성해 주실래요?

5. You need to fill out personal medical history form.

   개인 의학병력을 기입해 주셔야 합니다.

6. Would you please put on this gown?

   이 옷으로 갈아입으실래요?

7. You can change your clothes in the locker room.

   당신의 옷을 라커룸에서 갈아입으세요.

8. Rocker room is over there.

   라커룸은 저기에 있습니다.

9. Please, step on the height weight measurement machine.

   키, 체중 측정기에 올라가 서 주실래요?

10. You may step down.

    내려 오셔도 됩니다.

11. I am going to take your blood pressure.

당신의 혈압을 측정하겠습니다.

12. Would you please put your arm on the automatic blood pressure monitor?

자동 혈압계에 팔을 올려 주실래요?

13. You need to collect your midstream urine in this cup.

이 컵에 중간 소변을 받아주세요.

14. And return your urine specimen back.

그리고 소변 샘플을 가져와 주세요.

15. Have you brought your urine sample?

소변 샘플을 가져 오셨나요?

16. Put it on the table.

탁자 위에 놓아주세요.

17. You need to scoop some stool into container before you flush the toilet.

화장실 내리기 전 약간의 대변을 떠서 보관함에 담아 주세요.

18. Please bring it to us when you come next.

다음에 오실 때 저희들에게 가져다주세요.

19. We will have to do some tests such as EKG, X-ray, Ultrasonography.

심전도, 방사선 촬영, 초음파 등 검사를 할 것입니다.

20. We'll take a sample of your blood.

혈액을 채취할 것입니다.

21. All finished.

전부 끝났습니다.

22. You can get dressed now.

옷을 입으셔도 됩니다.

23. If you want to have additional optional tests, you have to

pay additional charges.

만약 추가 옵션 검사를 원하시면, 추가 비용을 지불하셔야 됩니다.

24. Do you want to make an appointment of government

subsidized health check up?

국가건강검진을 예약하시려고 하나요?

25. When would you like to make an appointment?

언제 예약하기를 원하시나요?

26. Are you available —?

—는 괜찮으신가요?

27. Come in at 8:00 AM.

아침 8시까지 오세요.

28. Make sure you don't eat anything for 8 hours before

check up.

검진 8시간 전에는 아무 것도 먹지 말아야 합니다.

29. If you have sedation endoscopy, your family

or friend have to escort you to your home.

만약 수면내시경을 받으면, 당신 가족이나 친구가 반드시

집까지 데려다 주어야 합니다.

제 3 부

43. 임상 검사 – 혈액 및 소변 검사
(Laboratory Test – Blood and Urine Sampling)

1. Please come in and have a seat.

   들어와 앉으세요.

2. We will have to do some laboratory tests on your blood.

   혈액 검사를 할 것입니다.

3. I'll take out some blood.

   혈액을 조금 뺄 것입니다.

4. Give me your arm.

   팔을 주세요.

5. Please roll up your sleeve.

   소매를 걷어 올리세요.

6. Can you make a fist? Clench your fist.

   주먹을 쥐어 주세요.

7. I am going to put a tourniquet on your arm to make the vein easier to find.

   정맥을 찾기 위해 팔에 압박고무를 감을 것입니다.

8. Hold your squeeze.

   그대로 쥐고 계세요.

9. That's fine.

   좋습니다.

10. You feel a little bit prick.

조금 따끔함을 느낄 것입니다.

11. Just relax. Take it easy.

편안하게 하세요.

12. Release your grip.

주먹을 푸세요.

13. I'll draw some blood through vessel.

혈관을 통해 피를 뽑겠습니다.

14. It'll hurt a bit.

약간 아플 것입니다.

15. There we go.

다 되어갑니다.

16. Is it painful?

아팠나요?

17. I got the blood that I needed.

필요한 혈액을 뽑았습니다.

18. We are done.

끝났습니다.

19. Hold this cotton and press down firmly.

이 솜을 가지고 꾹 누르세요.

20. Please take this paper cup.

이 종이컵을 받으세요.

21. Go to the bathroom and urinate in the cup.

화장실에 가서 컵에 소변을 누세요.

22. Discard the first flow and collect the midstream.

처음 소변 나오는 것은 버리고 중간 것을 받으세요.

23. Bring it back to us when you are done.

다 했으면 저희에게 가져다주세요.

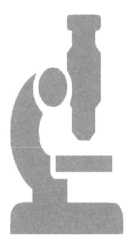

44. 방사선과 촬영실
(Radiology, X-ray Room)

1. Would you come over here?

   이곳으로 오실래요?

2. This place is the X-ray reception.

   이곳이 엑스레이 검사 접수처입니다.

3. Do you have an X-ray slip?

   방사선 처방전을 가지고 계시나요?

4. Is there any chance that you may be pregnant?

   임신 가능성은 없나요?

5. Please come this way.

   저를 따라 오세요.

6. Remove your top and put on this gown in the dressing
   room.

   탈의실에서 윗옷을 벗고 가운을 입으세요.

7. You need to take off your jewelry.

   귀금속들을 풀어야 합니다.

8. Stand over here against this plate.

   이곳에 서서 보드를 바라보세요.

9. Hold your hands on your back.

   손을 등 뒤에 대고 계세요.

10. Raise your arms up to shoulder height.

　팔을 어깨까지 올려주세요.

11. Take a deep breath and hold your breath.

　숨을 깊게 들이쉬고 참으세요.

12. Don't move.

　움직이지 마세요.

13. OK. You can breathe now.

　됐습니다. 숨을 쉬세요.

14. We need to take more X-rays.

　엑스레이 촬영을 더 해야 합니다.

15. Would you please lie down on the table?

　검사대에 올라가 누우실래요?

16. Take a deep breath and hold.

　숨을 깊게 들이쉬고 참으세요.

17. Breathe.

　숨을 내 쉬세요.

18. Try to keep as still as you can.

　가능한 가만히 계십시오.

19. Turn on your right side.

　오른쪽으로 도세요.

20. Turn on your left side.

　왼쪽으로 도세요.

21. Please Lie on your back.

반드시 누우세요.

22. All done.

다 끝났습니다.

23. You can put your clothes back on.

옷을 다시 입으셔도 됩니다.

24. Please don't forget to take all your belongings with you.

잊지 말고 당신의 물건들을 모두 챙겨가세요.

25. Please go to the outpatient's waiting place until

the X-rays are developed.

X-ray가 나올 때까지 외래 대기실에 가서 기다리세요.

26. The films will be developed soon.

필름들은 곧 현상될 것입니다.

27. Take care.

안녕히 가세요.

제 3 부

45. 청력 검사 (Hearing Test)

1. Would you please get in the booth?

   부스 안으로 들어가실래요?

2. Have a seat, please.

   의자에 앉으세요.

3. Audiometer will play a series of tones through headphones.

   청력계가 헤드폰을 통해 음을 계속 낼 것입니다.

4. The tones vary in pitch and loudness.

   음의 굵기나 크기는 다양합니다.

5. I will control the volume of a tone.

   음향 크기를 제가 조절 할 것입니다.

6. I will reduce its loudness until you can no longer hear it.

   당신이 소리를 듣지 못할 때까지 소리를 줄일 것입니다.

7. Then the tone will get louder until you can hear it again.

   그리고 다시 당신이 소리를 들을 때까지 커지게 할 것입니다.

8. You can signal each time you hear a tone by raising
   your hand.

   당신이 소리를 들을 때마다 당신의 손을 들어 주세요.

9. You can signal by pressing a button every time you hear
   a tone.

   당신이 소리를 들을 때마다 버튼을 눌러 주세요.

10. I will then repeat the test several times.

   몇 차례 검사를 더 할 것입니다.

11. Each ear is tested separately.

   각각의 귀를 다로 검사 할 것입니다.

12. Would you please wear headphones?

   헤드폰을 끼우실래요?

13. OK. You can remove the headphones.

   네. 헤드폰을 제거해 주세요.

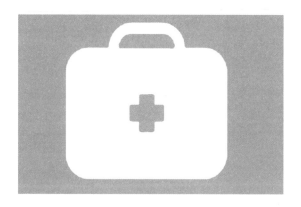

제 3 부

46. 시력 검사 (Eyesight Test)

1. I'll test your visual acuity.

   시력 검사를 하겠습니다.

2. The vision test (Visual acuity test) is always done
   at a distance of twenty feet.

   시력 검사는 항상 20피트 떨어져 검사합니다.

3. Stand on the line and read the eye chart.

   선 위에 서서 차트를 읽어주세요.

4. Look at straight ahead.

   앞을 똑바로 보세요.

5. I'll look into each eye.

   각 눈을 검사하겠습니다.

6. First, cover your left eye with paddle.

   가리개로 왼쪽 눈앞을 막으세요.

7. Can you see these letters?

   이 글자들이 보이나요?

8. Read from left to right.

   왼쪽에서 오른쪽으로 읽으세요.

9. OK. Cover your right eye.

   오른쪽을 가리세요.

10. Can you read this?

    이것을 읽을 수 있으세요?

11. You're finished.

끝났습니다.

12. Please follow my finger with your eyes without moving your head.

머리를 움직이지 말고 손가락을 따라 보세요.

13. We will examine your eyes.

눈을 검사하겠습니다.

14. Ophthalmoscopy requires dilating the pupils for the best view inside the eye.

검안경은 눈 안을 잘 보기 위해 동공을 확장시켜야 합니다.

15. I will place drops into your eyes to dilate the pupil.

동공을 열기 위해 안약을 눈 안에 떨어뜨릴 것입니다.

16. Getting your eyes dilated is painless.

눈이 확장되어도 통증은 없습니다.

17. Dilating drops works on iris muscle and opens the pupil.

동공을 확장시키는 약은 홍채에 작용해서 동공을 엽니다.

18. After the examination, your vision may remain blurred for several hours.

검사 후에 몇 시간 동안 눈이 희미해질 수 있습니다.

19. Bring a pair of dark sunglasses and a friend.

선글라스를 가져오고 친구를 데려 오세요.

20. Please sit here in front of the machine.

이 기계 앞으로 앉으세요.

제 3 부

21. Please rest your chin here and look straight ahead.

이곳에 턱을 대고 앞을 똑바로 보세요.

22. Keep your eyes open.

눈을 뜨세요.

23. Look at the marker on the screen.

스크린에 있는 표시를 보세요.

24. Look at the blinking light.

깜박거리는 불빛을 보세요.

25. The intraocular pressure is measured with a tonometer.

눈 안의 압력은 안압계로 측정합니다.

26. You will feel a soft pressure.

부드러운 압력을 느낄 것입니다.

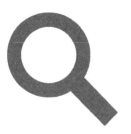

47. 심전도 검사 (EKG Test)

1. This is a painless procedure.

   이것은 아프지 않은 검사입니다.

2. Take off your shirt.

   서츠를 벗으세요.

3. Please, lie back on the bed.

   침대에 누우세요.

4. The test takes about 1 minute.

   검사는 1 분 정도 걸립니다.

5. A small amount of gel will be applied to the skin.

   약간의 젤이 피부에 발라질 것입니다.

6. Are you comfortable?

   괜찮으세요?

7. I am putting some gel on your wrist and ankle.

   손목과 발목에 젤을 바르겠습니다.

8. Just relax as much as you can.

   최대한 긴장을 푸세요.

9. I will attach EKG leads to your chest, both arms and legs.

   당신의 가슴과 팔, 다리에 EKG 선을 붙이겠습니다.

10. Don't move.

   움직이지 마세요.

11. I will check one more time.

한 번 더 검사하겠습니다.

12. It takes less than one minutes.

일 분도 안 걸립니다.

13. All finished.

다 끝났습니다.

14. You can get your clothes on.

옷을 입으세요.

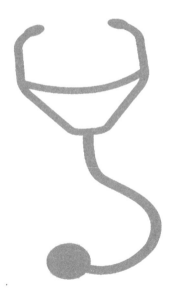

48. 초음파 검사 (Ultrasonography)

1. We will do Ultrasonography.

   초음파 검사를 할 것입니다.

2. Don't eat food exception of water for 8 hours prior to the examination.

   검사 8시간 전부터 물외에는 음식을 드시지 마세요.

3. Drink 1 liter of water one hour prior to the examination for the purpose of filling the bladder.

   방광을 채우기 위해 검사 1시간 전 1리터의 물을 마시세요.

4. Would you please lie down on the table?

   침대에 누우실래요?

5. Let your body relax.

   긴장을 푸세요.

6. Bend your knees.

   무릎을 구부려 주세요.

7. I will apply a gel to the surface of your body.

   당신의 몸에 젤을 바르겠습니다.

8. This won't hurt.

   이것은 아프지 않습니다.

9. You may feel coolness of the gel.

   젤이 차가울 수 있습니다.

제 3 부

10. OK. Lie on your left side.

됐습니다. 왼쪽으로 돌아누워 주세요.

11. OK. Lie on your right side.

됐습니다. 오른쪽으로 돌아누워 주세요?

12. All done.

다 끝났습니다.

13. Wipe off a gel on your body.

몸에 있는 젤을 닦으세요.

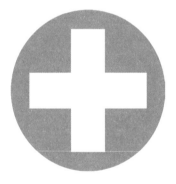

49. 상부 위장관 내시경
(Upper Gastrointestinal Endoscopy)

1. You will need to stop drinking and eating 8 hours before your endoscopy.

   내시경 전 8시간 전부터는 마시거나 먹으면 안 됩니다.

2. You will need to stop taking certain blood-thinning medication like aspirin for 1 week before your endoscopy.

   아스피린 같은 혈액응고 방지제는 내시경 일주일 전부터 끊으셔야 합니다.

3. An endoscopy tube will be inserted through your mouth.

   내시경 튜브가 입을 통해 들어갈 것입니다.

4. This may be a bit uncomfortable.

   이것은 약간 불편할 것입니다.

5. Endoscope will pass into the mouth and down the throat to the stomach and duodenum.

   내시경은 입을 통해 위와 십이지장까지 내려갑니다.

6. You'll feel it when it goes in.

   안으로 들어갈 때 느끼실 겁니다.

7. Doctor will take photos of ulcers or may remove a tiny piece of tissue.

   선생님이 궤양들 사진을 찍고 작은 조직을 떼어낼 수도 있습니다.

8. Lie on your left side on the bed.

   침대에 올라가 왼쪽으로 누워 주세요.

9. I will spray a local anesthetic to reduce discomfort

   and gagging.

   불편함이나 구토를 줄이기 위해 국소 마취제를 뿌리겠습니다.

10. You are lightly sedated during procedure.

    검사하는 동안 약간 진정제가 투여될 것입니다.

11. Please, hold this bite block and

    I'll give you a sedative to relax.

    자, 이제 이 내시경 마우스피스를 끼우시고,

    이제 진정제를 투여 하겠습니다.

12. You may feel mentally alert,

    but your reaction may be impaired.

    정신적으로는 깨어있을 수는 있으나 반응을 하기 힘들 것입니다.

13. Doctor will perform an endoscopy.

    의사선생님이 위 내시경 검사를 시작할 것입니다.

14. It won't hurt much.

    많이 아프지는 않을 것입니다.

15. Relax.

    긴장을 푸세요.

16. Doctor obtained small samples of the stomach tissue

    for biopsy.

    의사선생님이 조직검사를 위해 위의 조직 일부들을 떼었습니다.

242

17. You need to take the day off from work.

하루 동안은 일에서 쉬어야 합니다.

18. Your family or friend has to escort you to your home

because of sedation.

수면마취 때문에 가족이나 친구가 반드시 집까지 데려다

주어야 합니다.

19. Doctor will explain your results after a while.

선생님이 잠시 뒤 당신의 결과를 설명해 줄 것입니다.

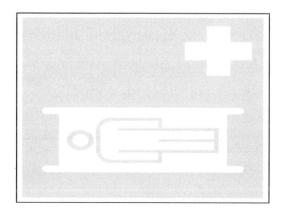

50. 대장내시경 (Colonoscopy)

1. Don't eat solid food with seeds or dark colors for at least
   2 days before colonoscopy.
   대장내시경 최소 2일 전부터는 씨가 있는 고형식이나
   진한 색의 음식은 드시지 마세요.

2. The night before a colonoscopy,
   you should have a liquid diet.
   대장내시경 검사 전날 저녁은 죽만 드셔야 합니다.

3. Evening before the colonoscopy,
   drink a liquid that will trigger bowel—clearing diarrhea.
   대장 내시경 전날 저녁 설사를 일으키는 용액을 마셔야 합니다.

3. You have to take half the laxative the night before the
   procedure and the other half about six hours before it.
   설사제를 시술 전날 밤에 절반 먹고, 시술 6시간 전에
   나머지 절반을 드셔야 합니다.

4. You need to dissolve the powder in 500cc water.
   500cc 물에 파우더를 녹여야 합니다.

5. Drink as much water as possible.
   가능한 물을 많이 드십시오.

6. We will use a long, flexible tube with camera to view
   the entire colon.
   대장 전체를 보기 위해 카메라가 달린 길고 잘 구부려지는

튜브를 씁니다.

7. You are lightly sedated before the exam.

   검사 전에 약간의 진정제가 투여될 것입니다.

8. Doctor will insert tube through the anus and rectum into
   the colon.

   선생님이 항문과 직장을 통해 내시경을 넣을 것입니다.

9. The procedure may cause a mild sensation of wanting
   to move the bowels and abdominal pressure.

   이 검사 도중 대변을 보고 싶거나 배에 힘을 줄 수 있습니다.

10. Sometimes we will fill the organs with air to get a better
    view.

    때론 더 잘 보기 위해 공기를 주입하기도 합니다.

11. The air may cause mild cramping.

    공기는 약간의 복통을 일으킬 수 있습니다.

12. If you feel any pain, just let us know.

    만약 아프면 저희에게 말해 주세요.

13. If an abnormality is seen, the doctor can remove a small
    piece of tissue for biopsy.

    만약 이상이 보이면 선생님이 조직 절편 일부를 떼어냅니다.

14. You may feel gassy and bloated after the procedure.

    당신은 시술 후 가스가 차서 배가 부른 것처럼 느낄 수 있습니다.

15. Caretaker has to escort you to your home.

    보호자가 반드시 집까지 데려다 주어야 합니다.

제 3 부

245

51. 전산화 단층촬영 및 자기공명 영상검사
(CT and MRI Examination)

1. CT scans emit more radiation than normal X-rays do.

   전산화 단층촬영은 X-선 촬영보다 방사선이 많이 방출됩니다.

2. But it is safe.

   그러나 안전합니다.

3. Special dye is injected into a vein before the scan.

   스캔 전에 특별한 약이 정맥 내로 주입됩니다.

4. The dye helps to show differences in the tissues.

   약이 조직에서의 다른 점을 보여줍니다.

5. Just let me know if you have any discomfort.

   불편한 점이 있으면 말해 주세요.

6. Please, lie down on the table?

   검사대에 올라가 누워주세요.

7. Take a deep breath and hold.

   숨을 깊게 들이마시고 참으세요.

8. OK. Breathe out.

   되었습니다. 숨을 내 쉬세요.

9. Magnetic Resonance Imaging is a way of looking inside the body without radiation.

   자기공명영상 장치는 방사선 피폭 없이 몸 안을 검사할 수 있는 방법입니다.

10. The exam uses radiowaves and a magnetic field to
create images of the soft tissues inside the body.
몸 안의 조직을 형상화시키기 위해 자기장을 이용합니다.

11. The complete exam takes 20 - 30 minutes.
검사는 20분에서 30분 걸립니다.

12. You can eat, drink, and take regularly prescribed
medications prior to the exam.
검사 전에 식사나 물, 처방된 약을 먹어도 됩니다.

13. All metallic objects on the body should be removed.
몸에 있는 금속은 제거되어야 합니다.

14. You will lie within the closed environment inside MRI.
당신은 MRI 안의 닫힌 곳에 누울 것입니다.

15. If you feel claustrophobic sensation, a mild sedative
will be given prior to MRI scan.
만약 당신이 밀실 공포증을 느낀다면, 약간의 진정제가
투여 될 것입니다.

16. You have to remain still during the exam.
검사하는 동안 움직이지 말아야 합니다.

17. Just relax your body.
몸을 편안하게 하십시오.

18. There is no pain, vibration, or unusual sensation.
고통이나 진동 같은 이상한 것을 느끼지 않습니다.

제 3 부

19. Relaxation is important during the procedure.

검사하는 동안 편안하게 하는 것이 중요합니다.

20. Please breath in and hold. OK. Breathe out.

숨을 들이쉬고 참으세요. 네. 숨을 쉬세요.

20. Breathe normally.

숨을 정상적으로 쉬세요.

21. We are all finished now.

이제 다 끝났습니다.

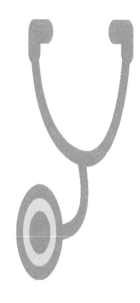

52. 조영제 사용
(Using the Contrast Medium)

1. Contrast enhanced scanning should be used for the differential diagnosis.
   감별진단을 위해서는 조영제 증강 검사가 필요합니다.

2. Contrast helps us visualize the condition of the disease.
   조영제가 질병의 상태를 더 잘 보여줍니다.

3. We will inject some amount of contrast into your vein.
   우리는 당신의 정맥으로 약간의 조영제를 투여할 것입니다.

4. Do you have any allergies?
   알러지가 있었던 적이 있습니까?

5. If you agree to this test, please sign your name in this consent form.
   만약 이 검사에 동의한다면 동의서에 사인을 해주세요.

6. I will perform a skin test for hypersensitivity.
   과민반응에 대한 피부검사를 할 것입니다.

7. I will scan you after a while.
   잠시 뒤 검사를 할 것입니다.

8. Would you like to lie on your back on this table?
   이곳 테이블에 올라와 누우실래요?

9. I will inject a contrast medium.
   조영제를 주사할 것입니다.

제 3 부

10. You may feel nausea or vomiting.

오심과 구토를 느낄 수가 있습니다.

11. If you feel any discomfort, just let me know.

불편함을 느끼시면 말씀해 주십시요.

12. You may experience an uncomfortable hot sensation.

아마도 뜨거운 듯한 불편함을 느낄 수도 있습니다.

13. Don't worry. It's not abnormal.

걱정 마세요. 이상한 것은 아닙니다.

14. It will fade after a little while.

잠시 뒤 약해집니다.

15. We are done.

다 되었습니다.

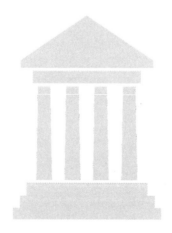

53. 접수처 (Reception Desk)

Very Useful Expressions

1. Can I help you?

    무엇을 도와드릴까요?

2. Do you want to check in?

    접수를 원하시나요?

3. What department do you want to check in?

    어느 과 접수를 원하십니까?

4. Is there a doctor you want to see?

    보시길 원하는 선생님이 계십니까?

5. Do you have a consultation request?

    진료의뢰서를 가지고 있나요?

6. What seems to be the problem?

    무슨 문제가 있으시죠?

7. You'd better make an appointment in A department.

    A과로 예약하시는 것이 좋을 것 같습니다.

8. Would you like to see Dr Lim? or Dr. Lee?

    임 선생님, 이 선생님 어느 분을 원하세요?

9. Do you want to see Dr. Kim?

    김 선생님을 뵙고 싶으신가요?

10. I'm sorry the doctor is not taking new patients.

죄송합니다. 선생님은 오늘 새로운 환자를 보시지 않습니다.

11. We'll call you if there are any cancellations.

취소가 있으면 연락을 드리겠습니다.

12. How about Dr. Lim?

임 선생님은 어떠세요?

13. I can schedule you with him.

그 분에게 예약을 하겠습니다.

14. 11 Am is best for you?

11시가 좋으신가요?

15. What's your name?

이름이 어떻게 되지요?

16. What's your last name?

성이 무엇이지요?

17. What's your first name?

이름은 무엇이지요?

18. Could you spell it out for me?

철자를 말해 줄래요?

19. What's your date of birth?

생일이 언제이지요?

20. Do you have medical insurance?

의료보험은 가지고 계십니까?

21. I would like to verify your identity.

당신의 신원을 확인하고 싶군요.

22. Do you have any identification card?

신분증이 있나요?

23. Could you fill out this form?

이 양식에 적어주세요.

24. What's your current address?

주소가 어떻게 되죠?

25. What's your telephone number?

전화번호가 어떻게 되지요?

26. We need you to sign this consent form on collecting
    your personal information.

개인 정보 동의서에 사인을 하셔야 합니다.

27. We need you to sign this paper.

서류에 사인이 필요합니다.

28. Please sign your name in this consent form.

이 동의서에 사인을 해주세요.

29. Your appointment is 10 O'clock.

당신의 예약은 10시입니다.

30. Please go there 5 minutes before your appointment time.

예약 시간 5분 전까지 그곳으로 가세요.

31. Did you finish your treatment?

진료를 다 마치셨나요?

32. The total charge is −won.

총비용이 −원입니다.

제 3 부

33. National health insurance doesn't pay for some items.

어떤 아이템은 국민 건강보험이 되지 않습니다.

34. Health insurance does not pay for all of your treatment costs.

건강보험은 치료비용을 모두 지급하지 않습니다.

35. How do you want to pay?

어떻게 지불을 하실 건가요?

36. By cash or credit card?

현금인가요? 신용카드인가요?

37. Please, sign your name here.

이곳에 사인을 해 주세요.

38. The clinic will be open from 9 AM.

진료는 9시에 시작됩니다.

39. The clinic will be closed from 5 PM.

진료는 5시부터 마감입니다.

40. Do you need to check in?

입원수속이 필요하신가요?

41. I can help you with the check in process.

입원 수속을 도와 드리겠습니다.

42. Which type of room do you prefer?

몇 인실을 원하시나요?

43. Single deluxe room? Two bedded room?
    4 bedded room? 6 bedded room?

1인실? 2인실? 4인실? 6인실?

44. If you want a private room, you may be expected to
    pay the additional fees.
    1인실을 원하시면 추가 비용이 발생합니다.

45. Do you want to check out?
    퇴원 수속을 원하시나요?

46. Do you want to have medical certificate and
    confirmation of hospitalization care?
    진단서와 입원확인서를 원하시나요?

47. The total cost is －.
    전부 비용이 －입니다.

48. How would you like to pay for it? Cash or card(charge)?
    어떻게 지불 하시겠습니까? 현금이나요 카드이나요?

49. I need your signature here.
    이곳에 사인이 필요합니다.

50. Here is your receipt.
    여기 영수증이 있습니다.

51. Parking will be free for up to 6 hours.
    주차장은 6시간까지 무료입니다.

제 3 부

Conversation

A : May I Help you?

무슨 일로 오셨죠?

P : I would like to see a doctor.

의사 선생님을 만나 뵙고 싶습니다.

A : Is this your first visit?

처음 방문을 하신 건가요?

P : Yes, it is.

네.

A : We need you to sign this consent form on collecting
your personal information.

개인 정보 동의서에 사인을 하셔야 합니다.

P : What's this?

이것이 무엇입니까?

A : This is a form that you agree to hospital's managing
your information for treating you.

이것은 당신을 치료하는데 필요한 정보를 다루는데
동의한다는 양식입니다.

And fill out this form.

그리고 이 양식도 적어 주세요.

P : OK.

알겠습니다.

A : Please tell me what your problem is.

무슨 문제가 있으시죠?

P : I have abdominal discomfort.

배 속이 불편합니다.

A : What did you eat last?

마지막으로 무엇을 드셨죠?

P : Nothing special.

별거 없습니다.

A : Who would you like to see?

어느 선생님을 원하세요?

P : I don't know any doctors here.

이곳 선생님들을 아무도 모릅니다.

A : I will arrange one for you.

한 명을 알아서 배정해 드릴게요.

P : Thank you.

감사합니다.

A : Wait a minute.

잠시 기다려 주세요.

제 3 부

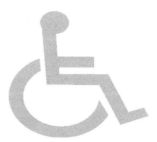

Extra Study

영어에 익숙하지 않을 때 쓸 수 있는 표현들

I can speak a bit of English.

저는 영어를 조금만 할 줄 압니다.

I am afraid you don't understand me.

제 말을 이해하지 못하신 것 같군요.

I can't express myself very well in English.

영어로 잘 표현하질 못합니다.

I can't understand very well in English.

영어를 잘 이해하지 못합니다.

Could you speak more slowly?

천천히 말씀해 주실래요?

Pardon me? Would you say that again?

뭐라고요? 다시 말해주실래요?

I can't think of it at the moment in English.

지금은 영어로 생각이 잘 안 나네요.

54. 진료 예약 (Making an appointment)

Very Useful Expressions

1. Sorry to have kept you waiting.

   기다리게 해서 죄송합니다.

2. Do you want to make an appointment?

   진료 예약을 원하십니까?

3. Who is your doctor?

   담당 선생님이 누구시죠?

4. Do you want to make an appointment with Dr. Kim?

   김 선생님에게 예약하시기를 원하나요?

5. What's your name?

   성함이 어떻게 되죠?

6. How do you spell it?

   철자가 어떻게 되지요?

7. What date do you want?

   어느 날짜를 원하시죠?

8. Which day is good for you?

   어느 날이 좋으시죠?

9. Let me see.

   잠깐 살펴보겠습니다.

10. I am afraid. Doctor is off on that day.

선생님이 그 날은 진료를 안 하시네요.

11. Do you think you can wait until -?

-날까지 기다리실 수 있으세요?

12. What time is good for you?

어느 시간이 좋으세요?

13. We have -, at 4 PM open.

-일 오후 4시가 비어있군요.

14. Will that be a good time?

괜찮습니까?

15. 3PM is filled.

3시는 예약이 다 되었습니다.

16. 3 : 20 PM open.

3시 20분이 비어있습니다.

17. Will you take it?

이것으로 예약을 하시겠습니까?

18. Your appointment is at 3 : 20 PM on -.

당신의 예약 시간은 -일 오후 3시 20분입니다.

Conversation

A : Hello, how may I help you?

안녕하세요. 무엇을 도와 드릴까요?

 Is this your first time to visit our hospital?

저희 병원에 처음 오셨습니까?

P : Yes it is.

네.

 I would like to make an appointment with Dr. Kim.

김 선생님에게 예약하려고 합니다.

A : What would you like to see him for?

무슨 문제로 그를 보려고 하세요?

P : I have a knee problem. It is aching.

무릎 문제입니다. 아파요.

A : Dr. Kim has openings twice per week.

김 선생님은 일주일에 2번 진료하십니다.

 Are you free on Tuesday or Thursday?

화요일이나 목요일 괜찮으세요?

P : I am free on Tuesday afternoon.

화요일 오후가 괜찮습니다.

A : When is good for you?

어느 시간이 좋으세요.

P : Any time will be fine.

어느 시간이든 좋습니다.

A : How about 2 PM?

오후 2시는 어떠세요.

P : It's good for me.

좋습니다.

A : I will schedule you for Tuesday at 2 PM.

화요일 오후 2시로 예약을 하겠습니다.

55. 예약 취소 및 변경
(Appointment Cancellation and Reschedule)

Very Useful Expressions

1. What day do you have appointment?

  약속하신 날짜가 언제신가요?

2. What time is it scheduled for?

  예약 시간이 언제이죠?

3. What's the reason for the cancellation/reschedule?

  최소나 변경을 원하시는 이유가 무엇입니까?

4. I will cancel it for you.

  취소를 하였습니다.

5. Do you reschedule your appointment?

  약속날짜를 변경해 드릴까요?

6. What day would you like to switch to?

  어느 날로 변경하시길 원하세요?

7. The doctor is not available at that time.

  그 시간에는 의사 선생님이 안 됩니다.

8. Can you make it at another time?

  다른 시간으로 하실래요?

9. What time would you like?

  어느 시간이 좋으세요?

10. I will put you down for that time.

그 시간으로 잡아드리겠습니다.

11. Your appointment has been changed to −.

당신의 약속은 −로 변경되었습니다.

12. If you arrive late, you may have to rebook to avoid delaying other patients.

늦게 오시면 다른 환자가 늦어지므로 다시 예약하셔야 합니다.

13. Thank you for calling to reschedule.

변경을 위해 전화를 주셔서 감사합니다.

14. We will see you then.

그때 뵙겠습니다.

예약환자가 오지 않은 경우

Hello, you have a doctor's appointment today?

여보세요, 오늘 진료 예약이십니다.

You missed your doctor's appointment.

진료 예약시간에 안 오셨네요.

Why didn't you come?

왜 안 오셨나요?

Did you forget your appointment?

예약을 잊으셨나요?

Can you come?

오실 수 있으세요?

264

Will you come to the hospital even if you are late?

늦었어도 병원에 오실래요?

If you couldn't come today, do you reschedule your

appointment?

오늘 못 오신다면 약속날짜를 변경해 드릴까요?

Conversation

A : Hello, How may I help you?

여보세요. 무엇을 도와 드릴까요?

P : I'd like to make an appointment with Dr. Kim.

김 선생님께 예약을 하고 싶습니다.

A : I am sorry. I have trouble hearing you.

죄송합니다. 잘 안 들리네요.

　Connection isn't clear.

연결이 깨끗하지가 않네요.

　Would you speak more loudly?

소리를 좀 더 크게 해 주실래요?

P : OK. I need to see the doctor.

알겠습니다. 의사 선생님에게 진료하려고 합니다.

A : Which doctor do you want to see?

어느 선생님을 보시길 원하시나요?

　Would you like to see Dr. Kim?

김 선생님을 보시길 원하시나요?

제 3 부

P : Yes.

네.

A : Hold one moment. Thanks for waiting.

잠깐만 기다려 주실래요? 기다려 주셔서 고맙습니다.

Doctor Kim is off today.

임 선생님은 오늘 오프입니다.

P : I was really hoping to see a doctor today.

오늘 진료를 하려고 생각했는데요?

A : What would you like to see him for?

무슨 증상으로 그를 만나려고 하시죠?

P: I have a headache problem.

두통이 있습니다.

A : How about seeing another doctor?

다른 의사 선생님을 보시는 것은 어떻습니까?

P: OK. No problem.

알겠습니다. 그렇게 하죠.

A : What's your names, please?

이름이 어떻게 되시지요?

P : Choi -.

최 - 입니다.

A : What's your date of birth?

생년월일이 어떻게 되지요?

P : -.

-입니다.

When is the doctor free?

선생님께서 언제 비어 있으시나요?

A : What time is good for you?

어느 시간이 좋으세요?

P : 3 o'clock PM.

오후 3시가 좋습니다.

A : Your appointment is at 3:00 PM.

당신의 예약 시간은 오후 3시입니다.

P : OK.

알겠습니다.

A : We'll see you at that time.

그때 뵙도록 하겠습니다.

 Have a good day.

좋은 하루 되십시오.

Extra Study

(If you don't speak English fluently － 영어를 잘 못할 경우)

I can't speak English well.

영어를 잘 못합니다.

Hold a moment, please.

잠시만 기다려 주세요.

I'd like to transfer to another person.

다른 사람에게 연결해 드리겠습니다.

56. 병원 안내 및 규칙 설명
(Information Desk)

Very Useful Expressions

1. What have you come here for?
   무슨 일로 오셨습니까?

2. Are you looking for someone?
   누구를 찾으세요?

3. She is in room 707 in the maternity ward.
   그녀는 산부인과 병동 707호에 있습니다.

4. Do you need directions?
   길을 알려 드릴까요?

5. The room is in the west wing.
   방은 서쪽 빌딩에 있습니다.

6. Take the elevator to the 7th floor and walk down the hall
   then make a right turn.
   승강기를 타고 7층으로 가서서 복도를 따라 가다가 우측으로
   도시면 됩니다.

7. You seem to be looking for someone.
   누군가를 찾고 있으신 것 같군요.

8. The patient was taken to ICU.
   환자는 중환자실로 가셨습니다.

9. Go straight down the hallway.

복도를 따라 쭉 가십시오.

10. Turn to the left at the corner.

모퉁이에서 왼쪽으로 도세요.

11. If you'd like to find patient, ask for help at the check in
desk.

만약 환자분을 찾으시려면 접수처에서 도움을 청하십시오.

12. The patient was discharged 2 hours ago.

환자는 2시간 전에 퇴원하셨습니다.

13. Patient is in the isolation ward.

환자분은 격리 병동에 있습니다.

14. We will take care of patient.

우리가 환자를 돌볼 것입니다.

15. Doctor is gonna explain it all to you when he gets here.

의사선생님이 이곳에 오면 당신에게 설명해 줄 것입니다.

16. You have to wait outside.

밖에서 기다리셔야 합니다.

17. Please wait in the waiting room.

대기실에서 기다려 주세요.

18. Sorry to have kept you waiting.

기다리게 해서 죄송합니다.

19. If you come with me, we'll get you admitted.

저를 따라 오시면 입원을 시켜 드리겠습니다.

제 3 부

269

20. Please, follow me.

저를 따라 오세요.

21. Come right this way.

이쪽으로 오세요.

22. Do you have any trouble?

무슨 일이 있으십니까?

23. Are you in a hurry?

급하시나요?

24. I'll show you to emergency room.

응급실로 안내해 드리겠습니다.

25. Would you come with me?

저를 따라 오실래요?

26. Follow the red line to emergency room.

빨간색을 따라 응급실로 가세요.

27. Family has to stay outside.

가족들은 저기 밖에서 기다려야 합니다.

28. You have to go with the kid to the waiting room.

어린이와 함께 대기실로 가 주서야 합니다.

29. Can I help you find something?

어디를 찾으세요?

30. There is a rest room in the west wing.

화장실은 서쪽 건물에 있습니다.

31. Down this hallway.

이 복도를 따라 가세요.

32. Rest room is around the corner.

화장실은 모퉁이에 있습니다.

33. The pharmacy is in the main hospital building.

약국은 병원 본부 건물 안에 있습니다.

34. Go through this door and turn right.

이 문을 지나 오른쪽으로 가세요.

35. You have to be mindful of your etiquette in hospital.

병원에서는 예의에 유념하셔야 합니다.

36. Please would you keep your voice down?

실례하지만 소리를 좀 낮추어 주실래요?

37. Smoking is not permitted in the hospital.

흡연은 병원에서 금지되어 있습니다.

38. You can't smoke here.

여기서는 담배를 못 피우십니다.

39. Do not leave your cell phone on in this area.

이 구역에서는 핸드폰을 켜 놓지 마세요.

40. You need to keep your things safely.

당신의 물건들을 안전하게 보관하셔야 합니다.

Conversation

A : Can I help you?

도와드릴까요?

P : I am not familiar with this area.

이곳을 잘 모릅니다.

How far is it to A from here?

여기에서 A까지는 얼마나 되죠?

Is it too far to walk there?

그곳까지 걸어가기는 너무 먼가요?

A : Yes, you'll have to take a bus.

네, 버스를 타야 될 것입니다.

P : Is there a bus to go to A?

A로 가는 버스가 있습니까?

A : Yes. Buses run every 10 minutes.

10분마다 버스가 있습니다.

P : Where do I take the bus?

버스를 어디서 타지요?

A : There is a bus stop right in front of this building.

이 건물 앞에 정류장이 있습니다.

P : Where can I wash my hands in this building?

이 빌딩에는 화장실이 어디 있습니까?

A : Down this corridor and to the right.

복도를 따라가다 보면 오른쪽에 있습니다.

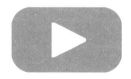

57. 화재 예방 및 화재시 대피
(Fire Prevention & Fire Evacuation)

Very Useful Expressions

1. If there is a fire, hospital emergency operations center will take care of it.

   만약 불이 나면 병원 비상대책 센터에서 조치를 취할 것입니다.

2. But everyone in the hospital must understand the escape plan.

   하지만 병원 안의 모든 사람들이 비상대피에 대해 알고 있어야 합니다.

3. We should be fully prepared for a real fire.

   실제 화재 상황에 대해 대비를 하여야 합니다.

4. We will make sure the escape routes are clear and doors can be opened easily.

   비상대피로가 확보되어 있고 문이 잘 열리는 지 확인할 것입니다.

5. When a smoke alarm sounds, get out immediately.

   화재경보가 울리면 즉시 밖으로 대피하십시오.

6. Your safety is paramount.

   여러분의 안전이 가장 중요합니다.

7. If the fire is small, confined, and not spreading, we have the appropriate type of extinguisher to fight the fire.

   만약 불이 작고 한정되어 있으면, 불을 끌만한 소화기가 있습니다.

제 3 부

8. We know the using method of the extinguisher.

우리는 소화기 사용 방법에 대해 알고 있습니다.

9. But if we can't take care of it, we will immediately report a fire to the fire station.

하지만 불을 끄기 힘들면 즉시 소방서에 화재를 알릴 것입니다.

10. We need to determine whether or not evacuation is required.

대피가 필요한 지 아닌 지 결정할 필요가 있습니다.

11. There is no immediate danger.

긴급한 위험은 없습니다.

12. Don't move patients, but begin to prepare for evacuation.

환자들을 옮기지는 마세요. 하지만 대피 준비는 하여야 합니다.

13. There is sufficient time for evacuation procedures.

대피할 시간이 충분히 있습니다.

14. Emergency move.

급히 피하세요.

15. Limited time to prepare is 5 to 6 minutes.

시간이 5-6분밖에 없어요.

16. Evacuate immediately
  or patients and staff may be dangerous.

즉시 대피하세요.

그렇지 않으면 환자나 직원들이 위험할 지도 모릅니다.

17. No time to prepare.

준비할 시간이 없어요.

274

18. Evacuate as quickly and safely as possible.

가능한 빨리 안전하게 대피하세요.

19. A full evacuation will not be required.

모두 대피할 필요는 없습니다.

20. There is a potential threat to patient safety.

환자들의 안전에 잠재적인 위험이 있습니다.

21. Partial evacuation will be required.

부분적인 대피가 필요할 것입니다.

22. Staffs need to be assigned multiple roles.

직원들이 여러 가지 일들을 담당해야 합니다.

23. It is important to identify the needs of serious patients.

중환자들에게 필요한 것들을 확인하는 것이 중요합니다.

24. Critical patients require specific life support equipment.

중환자들에게는 생명보조 장치들이 필요합니다.

25. In an immediate evacuation that is severely time sensitive,

the priority must be to get as many patients out as possible.

시간이 급박할 때, 가장 최선적인 방법은

가능한 한 많은 환자들을 밖으로 대피하는 것입니다.

26. But if time is critical, patients needing the most

assistance are the last to be moved.

하지만 아주 급박할 때는 가장 많은 도움이 필요한 환자가

가장 마지막으로 옮겨져야 합니다.

제 3 부

27. ICU patients may be moved after all of the general
    care units have been evacuated.

중환자실 환자들은 일반 병실 환자들이 모두 대피된 다음

옮겨져야 할지도 모릅니다.

Conversation

P : What's that sound?

저게 무슨 소리죠?

N : Don't worry. The fire alarm was activated by mistake.

걱정하지 마세요. 화재경보가 실수로 울렸습니다.

P : It's scary to think about a fire.

화재만 생각하면 무서워요.

  What can I do if there is a fire in the hospital?

병원에서 불이 나면 어떻게 하죠?

N : Once the fire alarm is triggered, our designated person will
    investigate the reason for the alarm and the possibility of
    a false alarm.

일단 화재경보가 울리면, 저희들 화재 담당자가 경보의 원인과

잘못 울렸는지 먼저 알아볼 것입니다.

P : What if there was a real fire?

정말로 불이 나면 어떻게 하죠?

N : We will identify the level of the threat and determine whether

the fire is a small one that can be suppressed or

whether evacuation is necessary.

위험 정도를 파악하여, 불을 쉽게 잡을 수 있는지,

아니면 대피해야 하는지 알아 볼 것입니다.

Every floor is equipped with fire extinguishers.

모든 층에 소화기들이 비치되어 있습니다.

We can quickly put out a small fire with fire extinguishers.

소화기들로 작은 불들은 끌 수 있을 것입니다.

P : How can I use the fire extinguisher?

소화기는 어떻게 사용하죠?

N : It's easy. At first pull the pin at the top of the extinguisher.

쉽습니다. 먼저 소화기 위의 핀을 잡아당기세요.

And aim at the base of the fire in order to put out the fire.

불을 끄려면 불이 난 아래쪽을 향하게 하셔야 합니다.

P : Sorry, I am not sure.

잘 모르겠는데요.

N : Squeeze the lever slowly.

레버를 천천히 쥐세요.

This will release the extinguishing agent.

그러면 소화액이 분사됩니다.

If the handle is released, the discharge will stop.

만약 레버를 놓으면 분사가 멈추어집니다.

Sweep from side to side, back and forth until the fire is completely out.

불이 꺼질 때까지 좌우, 앞뒤로 소화액을 뿌려주세요.

P : Oh, Now I see.

아 이제 알 것 같네요.

N : It's nothing. It's a piece of cake.

쉬워요. 누워 떡 먹기죠.

P : By the way, let me know the fire exit.

아무튼 비상구 좀 알려주세요.

N : OK. There are two emergency exits on every floor.

모든 층에는 비상구가 2곳이 있습니다.

I will show you all possible exits and escape routes.

가능한 비상구를 다 알려주겠습니다.

(In Case of Fire, 불이 난 경우)

P : Fire! Someone has sounded the alarm.

불이야! 누가 화재경보기를 울렸네요.

N : In the event of accidental small fires, we can put out the fire.

작은 불이 난 경우에는 불을 끌 수 있습니다.

Staff members know how to use the fire extinguisher.

병원 직원들이 소화기 사용법을 알고 있습니다.

P : Everyone else is leaving the area.

모두가 대피하고 있어요.

Someone has called the fire department.

누가 소방서에 전화했습니다.

N : Don't be afraid.

놀라지 마십시오.

We put out a fire.

불을 껐습니다.

P : What a relief.

다행이네요.

If suppression the fire is failed, how do we act?

만약 불을 끄는 것이 실패하면 우리는 어떻게 해야 하죠?

N : We have to evacuate the all patients, visitors, and staff

out of dangerous facilities as safely as possible.

모든 환자들과, 방문객, 직원들을 가능한 안전하게 위험한

지역에서 대피시킬 것입니다.

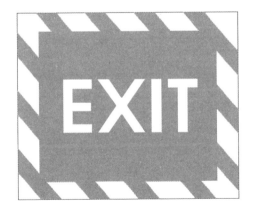

I am proud of myself
and all the progress I continue to make.

자신의 마음을 진취적이고
긍정적으로 바꾸어 주는 좋은 문구들

Think globally, act locally.

Manage yourself and time, and then lead others.

Be the self-motivated people & Enjoy your work.

Try to keep good constitution.

Feel bio-energy and whole connected world.

Freedom has many different faces.

Enjoy commonality and ordinary life.

Try to fuse the technology and the liberal arts.

Love has unlimited ways.

Do your best and never give up.

Our thoughts become things.

Try to be more intelligent and brilliant.

Burst inspiration & Inspire next.

Put focus on people relationship.

Proceed to next goal.

Keep smiling and keep yourself happy.

Keep emotionally healthy.

Insightful thinking and methodical approach.

Focus on what you are paying attention to.

Make no distinction and use positive term.

Turn idea into reality.

Become intensely aware of what is happening in this moment.

Respect privacy and individuality.

Patience is a virtue.

Be a warm hearted person.

Be diligent and live in the moment.

Let it be and let it go.

No waste time. Time is of the essence.

Keep healthy and lively condition.

Simple is better.

Enjoy working out and keep in shape.

No pain, no gain.

Love draws love.

Rest in peace and act in passion.

Free from any bias.

Just be yourself.

Be a citizen of the world.

Don't attach to desire.

Get organized to increase the power of creation.

More understanding needed, not more persuasion.

Keep up-to-date with the latest thinking.

Feel the social change and use social stream.

Passion for knowledge and truth.

Gather information and become more adaptive.

Open your mind and Level with others.

Don't wander off in the distractions of the past and future.

Building self confidence is the heart of self development.

There is nothing you can do to change a past moment.

Have a global mind.

Feel whole life energy and enjoy your life.

Follow your heart and humanity.

Getting ready is the secret of success.

Be in fashion and try to be confident.

Be one whom nobody can imitate.

Experience is the best teacher.

A sound mind in a sound body.

Step by step one goes very far.

Have a general idea of what is going on in the world.

Focus on positive thoughts and forward thinking mind.

Feel and understand the mainstream of society and modern life.

Creative thoughts and works impact the world.

Constancy of purpose achieves the impossible.

Power is in your thoughts.

Enjoy liberal mind.

Go confidently in the direction of your dreams.

Feeling happiness make you healthy.

Expectation is the powerful attractive force.

Your love attracts positive power.

Kindness is the golden chain.

Develop your general knowledge and ability to think.

Decide your fate for yourself.

Great capacity for patience and understanding.

Everything has the value, but not everyone sees it.

If you don't aim high, you will never hit high.

Happiness is a perfume you cannot pour on others

without getting a few drops on yourself.

Spirituality is not about what you're doing,

it's about what you're being.

Great minds think alike.

It all depends on how we look at things,

and not how they are in themselves.

We were given two ears but only one mouth.

This is because God knows that

listening is twice as hard as talking.

The more curious you are,

the more possibilities you will open throughout your lifetime.

간호영어 병원영어

1판 1쇄 2017년 2월 20일

2쇄 2021년 7월 05일

지은이 / 임창석

펴낸이 / 임준형

출판사 / 아시아 북스

등록 / 2015년 8월 5일 제 2015 – 000065 호

주소 / 서울시 송파구 문정동 법원로55 송파아이파크 오피스텔 C동 903호

전화 / 02-407-9091

팩스 / 02-407-9091

E-mail : Asiabooks@naver.com

저자와의 계약에 의해 아시아 북스 출판사에서 발행합니다.

ISBN 979-11-955956-4-8 (93510)